NO MR FAT GUY

THE Nutrition and Fitness Programme for Men!

Jonathon Savill and Richard Smedley

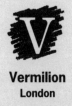

Vermilion
London

1 3 5 7 9 10 8 6 4 2

First published in the United Kingdom in 1998 by Vermilion
This new edition published in 2000 by Vermilion
an imprint of Ebury Press
Random House
20 Vauxhall Bridge Road
London SW1V 2SA

Random House Australia (Pty) Limited
20 Alfred Street, Milsons Point, Sydney,
New South Wales 2061, Australia

Random House New Zealand Limited
18 Poland Road, Glenfield,
Auckland 10, New Zealand

Random House South Africa (Pty) Limited
Endulini, 5A Jubilee Road,
Parktown 2193, South Africa

Random House UK Limited Reg. No. 954009

A CIP catalogue record for this book is available from the British Library

ISBN: 0 09 182595 4

Printed and bound in Great Britain by
Cox & Wyman, Reading, Berks

Contents

Acknowledgements

This book was written during the time that Richard and I were going about our separate working lives. It was added to in Norway, Thailand, America (three times), Denmark, Russia, Croatia, Germany, Holland, Italy, Spain and South Africa.

Jonathon's thanks

During the course of the whole adventure many people lent help and encouragement, each adding strength from their own expertise. More or less in order they are: Judy, Jamie and Toby Savill, for being my family and my friends too. Stephen Ferns, editor (at that time) of the health section of *GQ*. Richard, for being good under difficult circumstances. Chris Nickson helped to find Laura, without whom . . . . Ruth Nicholas and Chris Nickson nagged me lots and Norman Hartley was my best friend – after Judy, of course. Chris Coates, Tony Lennon, the Red Devils, Victor Osborne, and Mike Popham all gave me encouragement right from the start and for that I will always be grateful. Danny Perry from Sting's tour marvelled at the enormity of writing this book and made me finally realize just how big the task was. Thanks too to Levi jeans, for making 34-inch waists.

Richard's thanks

I too would like to thank Stephen Ferns, but I'd also like to kill him for introducing me to Jonathon. Laura has been a good friend to us. Abner Stein accepted us at face value and even bought us lunch. Lance and Sadie and Lizzie from next door to Jonathon all helped. Jonathon worked out OK as a team, which surprised us both. Maria was my girlfriend and, who knows, she might be again now I've finished the book. Thanks also to Joanna at Ebury for being elastic about the deadlines.

Introduction

The book is not just about getting thin, it's about getting to your correct weight, being physically fitter and feeling good about yourself. It's about putting you in control of your body. Scary, huh?

It's not a diet. A diet is a temporary thing you do and then stop. A diet is something you fail at. Being on a diet is like being on a motorway: you're either on it or you're lost on a side road. What this book does is help you to follow a healthy eating plan. It's not dogmatic. When you follow it, you keep moving overall in the right direction, and if you lose your way for a moment you have the control and the knowledge to come back on line. And you'll want to. There's no pass or fail; it's not an exam. Call it continuous assessment. It's your body and all you've got to do is to really like it.

This is about self-image; it will help you to feel better about yourself. If you're happy being fat, then put the book down and go buy a novel. If you're not happy about being fat, this is the book for you. I'm human, just like you, so I know how hard it can be to do this stuff.

I started out weighing nearly 120 kg (18 stone 10 lb). I was 42 years old with two children and a big mortgage. I don't have loads of money. I had high blood pressure and if I moved my head quickly I could see the Grim Reaper out of the corner of my eye. I was waiting for a heart attack to happen. In short, I am no different from many other people. I don't expect you to do 500 press-ups immediately; I couldn't then and I can't now.

But you have to want to get to your correct weight. I mean really want to. It's no good saying 'Well, that's it, I've failed. I may as well give up.' If you suddenly make a break for the cake, start eating properly again as soon as you can. If you find yourself in a social situation where the food is unhealthy, eat the least harmful thing and then go back to proper eating as soon as possible.

Most people slide into diets reluctantly. They act as though they are being forced to leave their loved ones, but will return as soon as they can – 'Farewell, doughnuts, I am going into the dark country, but I'll be back, I'll be back.' The fact is that what we consider to be healthy food actually tastes nicer than the bad stuff we love so much. Dieting has connotations of not eating normally. As soon as you are thin, you go back to getting fat again. This book will teach you how to eat healthily as the norm, and to control how your body looks. It's a food philosophy.

I've discovered that so-called 'proper food' makes you feel better. Be honest, when you're fat don't you dread some skinny shop assistant sneering at you? I had a 106.5-cm (42-inch) waistline at the beginning of this programme, and I recently had to send back a pair of trousers with a 91.5-cm (36-inch) waist I'd ordered because they were too big. I'll say that again: they were *too big*! Yessss.

As I got thinner and exercised more, I discovered that I actually had a pretty fast metabolism and now I can, within reason, eat more or less what I want to. But, oddly, I really don't want to eat all the rubbish that I ate before.

When you start a diet, some of your friends will try to stop you. They'll poke fun at you and they'll make a big point of ostracizing you for not eating the same as them or not drinking loads of alcohol. And the ones who make the most fuss or noise will either be the fattest ones, or the ones with fat partners. 'Oh, I forgot you can't drink any more, can you?' was the constant refrain of one friend. The same friend was fascinated with my weight loss later and kept complimenting me on my figure. Another friend stared at me blearily through the bottom of a vodka bottle. 'You'll soon get back to reality,' he said.

Another assumption people make is that you'll lose a lot of weight, and then put it all on again. People say to me, after I lost nearly 25.5 kilos (4 stone), and over 20 cm (8 inches) off my waist, achieved perfect blood pressure and acquired a built-in personal turbo-charger, 'Are you going back?' Yeah, right.

Right, you've made it through so far. You're strong enough for this. There is no unique secret. Work and will-power will get you thin. 'Terrific!' I hear you cry as you toss the paperback into the waste-disposal unit, '£6.99 down the drain.' But wait – we can help you. We just can't magic the fat away. What we can do is to explain a bit about how your body works and how you can eat maybe even more than you're eating now and still get thin. This book is about using a combination of food control and exercise to achieve the shape you want.

Basically, you choose what shape you are every time you eat something. The person with the six-pack stomach didn't get it through drinking six-packs. If you eat a lot of cream cakes you will get fatter. Fact. A banana is better for you and tastes just as sweet after a while. Now, in case you think I am being Mr Smug Bastard, I have probably eaten more sticky buns than anyone else in England. I ate so much Indian food that people thought I was single-handedly trying to reclaim the Raj.

I drank on average six cans of cider every night. It's not that I can't drink now, it's just that the idea of getting drunk every night no longer has the same appeal. It's not that you can't drink. You can. You can eat chips when you want to. But the major change I made is that I don't want to any more. Sometimes I crack, of course, but I no longer consistently eat things that are patently bad for me on a regular basis. I still love chocolate, but limit myself to a couple of squares every now and again instead of a whole bar every day. I still feel like I did something awful, and I still get the aftertaste, but I've cheated by 100 calories instead of 600.

One thing that eating correctly does do is let you enjoy food and drink again. No, eating healthily doesn't stop you enjoying things. I enjoy wine more than I ever did when I was drinking it regularly. Now I drink a glass, or maybe two glasses, of wine two or three nights a week. It's Nirvana, I can taste every grape and it's delicious. I drink it slowly; I no longer throw it down my neck. I don't drink wine when I'm thirsty. I drink it only to enjoy it and I stop drinking while I'm still enjoying it.

A lot of our attitudes towards food are wrong. For example, children are routinely made to eat more than they want to. 'Eat up, dear, you're not leaving the table till your plate's empty.' Why? There's no shortage of food any more. This attitude is the leftover of a wartime-rationing mentality.

Also, people make a kind of taste Hiroshima with sometimes literally dozens of conflicting tastes. Take a chicken sandwich. A healthy chicken sandwich consists of brown bread, chicken breast, salad and maybe lemon juice. It's simple and delicious. Now add loads of butter and mayonnaise and make the sandwich on white bread. Suddenly you have a gloopy mess, the white bread goes soggy, the whole thing dribbles all over your clothes, and the calorie content has trebled. And it doesn't taste any nicer.

I did have a lot of help in getting fit, but before I talk about how I lost the weight I want to look at the reasons why I gained it in the first place. I quit smoking at 30. At the time I had a 91.5-cm (36-inch) waist. I know that because in my closet sat a load of clothes that I am able to more or less date and I know their waist sizes. My wardrobe was a kind of black museum to fatness, loads of clothes that I was never going to wear again. Now I've come down the scale I've thrown them all away. If I get fatter I'll I have to go naked. Everything fits me now. By the time I was 32, my waist was a steady 96.5 cm (38 inches). By the age of 36 my waist was 101.5 cm (40 inches), and at 42 I was heading out to 107-cm (42-inch) waist country.

Coming down from that waist measurement to 86 cm (34 inches), where I am now, took a little over twelve weeks. OK, now you're building up your excuses. 'I haven't got time to get fit.' Actually, the four hours I spent slumped in front of the television every day divided into two hours for exercise and two more hours playing with the kids. 'I could never lose weight that fast.' Maybe you can't, and in fact I lost mine under strict supervision.

What we are doing in this book is showing you a track. How far you follow it is up to you. What I can tell you is that it's worth it. I've gone a long way down it and so far it has given me immense pleasure and repaid me every step of the way. Richard, my trainer, has been fit all his life. He taught me and taught me well, but if he says, 'This is how you do it,' you think, 'Yeah, that's easy for you to say.' I was a slob. I am not Richard Gere, God knows, but I look as good as I can. And I feel as good as I could, too. That is what we want to teach you.

Those exercises that show super-models lying on a beach in Hawaii don't matter a bean to folks like us, do they? What we're saying to you is 'Be the best you can.' You'll start by getting a bit better and then it will snowball. You'll find yourself rolling with it and building up speed.

The fact is that if you're fat, it's partly because you're eating too much. Why? Well, in my case it was a comfort thing. I gradually increased the amount I needed to make myself happy. I ate my food and then snuffled round the table eating other people's food. One more bread roll than anyone else. I never gave serious thought to what I ate. Actually I always thought about what I ate, but I was always planning one meal before I finished another. Places began to have food associations. Wareham in Dorset had the greatest cream cakes, other places great Indian restaurants, and so on.

As you get thinner, other comforters replace what food used to give you. I remember the first time my trousers felt looser. After a couple of weeks, I started to need a belt. Then the belt needed to be tighter. And then I needed tighter trousers. Believe me, no food 'high' can replace that feeling. People use food to comfort themselves because they had a bad day or because they failed at something.

As you get fitter, life gets easier. Funnily enough, money becomes less important. People buy things to make them feel better. When I was fat, I often bought things I didn't need, like extra cameras. Then I had to pay for them. More pressure. When you're fit, you have fewer problems. You become more capable somehow. Things don't upset you so much.

Food is fuel. It's strangely liberating to lessen its importance in your life. You eat only when you're hungry. When you go to the supermarket you can look in a trolley and know what the person pushing it will look like before you look at them. So here's a tip. Before you go shopping try to work out how you would like to look, and make your trolley reflect that. The way we sometimes eat in England can be a bad idea. For example, on Saturday night you drink 18 pints of lager, go out for a curry, then go home and fall asleep on the sofa. Where do you think that energy is going to go? Right, it's going to turn to fat. It's the only place that it can go, you can't use it for running when you're asleep.

So now we've lined up the new you on the runway. We've checked for any loose bits that may fall off on the journey. We've made sure that the fuel you take on will be pure. And you're going to exercise. When I started this diet I couldn't run 5 metres/yards. I'm not Linford Christie now, but I can run on a treadmill for 40 minutes and then row for another 20. And, extraordinarily, I've discovered that I like bike-riding.

The idea of getting up for exercise is abhorrent to almost any human being. Getting on a bicycle first thing on a cold morning is horrible. But I took up cycling only because I hated it less than other forms of exercise, but now I find that once I'm on the bike I actually enjoy it. For a start, it's time I can use to shut my mind off from everything else, or to think about something I don't have time to think about later in the day. I found that it made me feel virtuous too, and I started smiling at people who were struggling into the world after a heavy breakfast. Also, you notice things more when you're exercising.

You will find that, as you get a bit fitter, you will feel younger. You can wear clothes that look like they did in the catalogue or on the rail in the shop. You can buy mail-order clothing knowing it will fit you. This is very liberating. It allows you to feel good about yourself. And that's what we want you to achieve. Just that: feeling good about you.

Everything you learned to do you learned a bit at a time. The same applies to becoming fit and healthy. We agree that the longest journey begins with a single step. In this case it begins with a single book.

1
Why Change?

When human beings stopped being amoebas and crawled on to dry land, their first and almost only priority was to survive. The world was a different place. In order to survive, they needed shelter, food and fire. Life was tough and good physical abilities were essential. In some less-developed parts of the world they still are, of course.

In earlier ages, most of man's achievements were directly linked to his physical abilities. To run, walk, build, hunt, and kill, he had only one essential tool: his body. Unless it was in top shape, he wouldn't survive, because life was stripped to its bare essentials. His way of life kept him in good shape and ensured he could get the most from his body. People who were in less than perfect shape would almost certainly die, just as animals in the wild do now.

The world has evolved and different skills are now needed. Imagine what use the animal kingdom would have for a chartered accountant or a foreign-exchange dealer. We are developing as a race who no longer need to be fit to survive. We can get a Ferrari instead of a perfect physique. Instead of running or walking, we drive, or take a bus or a taxi. If we want to eat, we don't pick up a spear – we pick up a credit card. Even our entertainment is sofa-based.

In addition our requirements are getting bigger and more complicated all the time, including silly things like electric windows. Not so long ago they were a luxury, now almost every car has them. It's the same with food. We no longer accept seasons in our food-buying. So, if you want strawberries in December you can get them – at a price. This miracle of availability is partly the result of a wonderful and efficient transport system, but it has also been gained by using chemicals to make our food last longer.

The food we eat is very complicated in its content and preparation, through which it loses much of the natural goodness it contains. We have become used to nutrition being a vast and elaborate process. It seems absurd that we must now pay a great deal more for food that has not been treated or touched by chemicals. Imagine trying to explain the concept of expensive organic food to someone in the Third World. 'It goes like this: we pay loads extra for vegetables with the dirt still on them', or slimming food. I remember being in Romania just after the revolution, when people were literally starving. Any food they could get was disgusting. A packet of slimming soup had somehow found its way into the mountain of food that we were delivering to the country as volunteer aid workers. I explained to one of the Romanian hostel workers the concept of slimming food. 'You mean that you pay extra for food without any calories? What vanity.'

It is only a relatively small amount of societies that regard calories as harmful. In many situations or cultures, it is essential to take in as many calories as possible. Someone digging the road will use up about 3500 calories, but Royal Marines training in the Arctic Circle have their calorific intake raised to around 8000 every day. They eat boiled sweets, Mars bars and a pudding at every meal. A fatty's dream.

The point is that calories are not bad; we need them. Nor is food our enemy, although certain types of food do us more harm than good. It's the fact that we are largely a sofa-based society eating like Boston whalers which is making us fatter as a race.

We may be better off living in Croydon and eating hamburgers than we would be living in a cave and eating raw dinosaur, but because we exert ourselves less than our prehistoric ancestors, we're generally less efficient at using up those calories. Our food also has fertilizers, hormones, growth stimulants and preservatives built in. Add to that time-watching, stress and money worries, and we have the perfect recipe for a heart attack. Most of us have become so obsessed with everything else in our lives that we have lost touch with our bodies, are overweight and neglect our health.

There's our excuse: it's not us, it's the world we live in. It's the availability of easy-to-eat junk-food snacks in every garage, station and corner shop in the land. But the solution lies with us. Somehow we've convinced ourselves that because of the lives that we lead we can't do anything about it. Healthy eating and exercise are something we can't make time to do. Wrong. These are things we can't live without.

Why do we need to be fit and healthy? Does it improve our chances of finishing that essay/report/synopsis by Friday? Will willing members of the opposite sex suddenly throw themselves at me?

(Actually, they might.) When we talk about fitness, we don't mean running marathons every day, but achieving a moderate level of fitness which in turn will lead to good health. The difference between exercising correctly three times a week for, say, an hour each time and exercising six times a week for two hours is not that great in terms of getting healthy. The major difference is the one between taking a reasonable amount of exercise and none at all.

So what's stopping you? Let's look at some of the reasons that people give for being unable – or unwilling – to eat better or get fitter. (There may even be some here that you haven't thought of.)

- I'm much too busy. I just couldn't make time to go to the gym.
- My family hardly ever see me as it is. If I start getting fit they'll see even less of me.
- I'm naturally big-boned.
- Fitness is boring and people who do exercise are nerds.
- Who wants to be seen in a mauve leotard?
- People who don't drink are no fun.
- It's not fair on my kids.

Here is the other side of the coin:

- If you get fit, you feel better.
- Your clothes will look better on you.
- Your self-respect will grow.
- Your kids will be proud of you and they'll have a more active parent to play with.
- Your chances of the following are much reduced: heart disease, lung cancer, back problems, blood pressure, osteoporosis.
- You will have more energy.
- You will see the world in a more positive light.
- Being fit reduces stress.
- You may actually get to have more free time, because you spend less time sitting on the sofa watching television.

There is a general feeling of well-being when you are fit. Being unfit is a bit like driving an old banger down the motorway. Your chances of making it to the end are probably OK, but you worry all the time. If you are driving a good car down the motorway the possibility of breaking down never occurs to you; your brakes are better, so your chances of avoiding a crash are that much greater. Old cars *do* make it down to the end of the motorway, and you sometimes see expensive brand new cars on the hard shoulder, but statistically your chances are better in a machine in good condition. The same is true of your body on life's racetrack.

When you are fit you spend less time looking for other things to improve your life. I have three friends who own new Ferraris. Two of them are in therapy and the other one ought to be. You can't replace the core of your existence with objects.

More and more people in this country are overweight today. I'm not asking you to start jogging at once, but you could begin by having a good look at yourself in the mirror. If you have kids, go to the park with them or take them cycling. One friend of mine has a nine-year-old son and he has never taken him cycling or swimming. So the chances of the son growing up to be super-fit are minimal, to say the least.

Remember that what you do affects your children too. If you smoke, your children are more likely to be smokers. Fact. If you eat masses of fatty food, your kids will probably end up looking like little porkers as well. Look at the fat parents in the supermarket then check out their kids. See?

How do you know if you're too fat? The fact that you've bought the book suggests that you think you are. You may have an idea of how you would like to look. It's probably thinner than you need to be and may be thinner than you'll get. But you're going in the right direction if you have a go.

Statistically the odds are against you as well. Obesity is rising at an alarming rate all over the Western world. You could be just another statistic. Or you could read this book and make it work for you. Your choice.

2
Mind-set and Motivation

So you're on the starting block and you've got the best of intentions. You've got motivation, will-power and a goal. So why do we nearly all fail? Because our methods of achieving our goals are often poor and this in turn decreases our chances of success.

Here are some ideas developed by sports psychologists that will help you approach and conduct your training in an intelligent and positive way. Read them carefully because they will help you succeed by bringing a realistic perspective to the task ahead of you.

Set realistic, attainable goals

This is the bit that keeps you motivated or makes your plans go up in smoke. It is vital to set realistic goals right at the start, otherwise you will fail and go back to your old comforters. If you find yourself failing, it's because you've probably been too hard on yourself at the beginning. Change your plans if you're not achieving your targets. Be easier on yourself if you have to. If you run, set a distance that you know you can achieve, albeit with some effort. Tell yourself that you can't fail, you can only digress. Don't be too easy on yourself, either. There's no point in saying 'OK, I'll lose a few grams and then go for a curry.' You've got to work at it. But it's worth it.

Set specific goals

If you say 'I'll get a bit thinner and look a bit better,' you never will. But if you say 'I'll lose 10 kilos, or keep going till I can run for 5 kilometres,' and you try hard, you probably will achieve your goal one day.

When you set your goals, don't write a novel. Make them short and memorable so that you can repeat them to yourself through gritted teeth when you're running through the woods in the rain.

Make them relate to each other, too. If your main priority is simply to get in better shape, one related goal could be to decrease your resting heart rate from 75 to 65 BPM (beats per minute). This means that your heart won't work as hard. You may also want to bring your blood pressure down to 125/70 (see the next chapter for what this will mean for you). You may also want to reduce your body fat percentage, from 25 per cent down to 18 per cent, for example.

Express goals positively

What this advice means is that if you set your goals thinking 'I hope I don't overeat' or 'I hope I don't miss training this week,' you will definitely fail. Don't think negatively.

Saying 'I will go training' or 'I will finish this circuit/run' shows a positive attitude and you'll find it more effective.

Chop up big goals into small ones

Oy, you on the sofa. Yes, that's right, you with the chips. If you say 'I'll run a marathon,' it's so silly that you reach for another can of lager, shake your head and the whole thing's finished. But if you start off wanting to run to the corner to get your lager, it's a start.

Put another way: if you work up to your goal in realistic steps you will find success. So you can set a long-term goal, such as running a marathon. Then break it up into small, achievable steps. 'OK, I'll run 5 kilometres in a set time.' Then you're on your way.

Be flexible

Don't give up if you fail. This is not an exam; think of it as continuous assessment. If you fail to make an exercise session because you had to do something important, or even because you were just too idle, make it up another way on another day.

If you go screaming mad and become the creature that ate the planet, finish the chip orgy and then go back to real life. Eat better at the next meal. This is not diet land, this is real life, and you will fail quite often. But you must make sure that when you do you get back on track. I used to be fat and now I'm thin. I'm not Superman.

The way it's done sometimes involves failing and then feeling guilty. When I felt guilty, I backstepped to the good guys' line.

If you keep failing, you must adjust your goals so that they work for you.

Keep track of your objectives

It's good to know how you're doing. Although I really wanted to write this book, I kept putting it off until the last minute. So I made a little computer spreadsheet that told me what percentage of the typescript I'd completed. Every time I finished 1000 words, I put it on the spreadsheet and watched the percentages jump. Soon I was bashing away 1000 words just for the pleasure of it and the book got finished faster. I didn't work any harder than I would have otherwise, but by tracking it I saw myself climbing the ladder.

I was the same when I was losing weight. I weighed myself every week and took real pleasure in watching every gram go. I also set myself landmarks, such as 'Crack 108 kilos (17 stone)' or 'Lose two kilos (4½ lb)'. Each goal met is a major triumph and gives you the momentum to go for the next one. When you're failing at something, each new obstacle is like a punch; it throws you back on to the ropes and makes it harder for you to recover.

Think 'I am an active person'

I forced myself to feel fit right from the start. By that I mean I forced myself from the beginning to take the active rather than the slothful choices in my everyday life. These included walking quickly up and down the platform when waiting for a train; taking my kids to the park to play; running up escalators in the underground; cycling or walking to appointments instead of tubing it or going by car. I also joined a cheap gym and it cost per session the same as a can of lager. All these activities are open to everyone and it really takes very little mind-set to make them happen. You'll be surprised how it can affect the way you feel about yourself. Go for it.

As we said at the beginning of this book, you've got to *want* to get fit. You know at least 20 people who smoke and you know at least three who have given up smoking. Why did the three succeed when the others all failed? Because they *wanted* to succeed.

It may sound like that awful mind-set guru stuff, but your basic need is for the wish to improve yourself. Once you got it, you're there. This book can't give you will-power, but it can point out good reasons to develop it and show you the path once you've got it. (Failing that, it will prop up a wonky table-leg for years to come.) It can help you if you really want to succeed. And you do, don't you?

3
Stress

Stress is part of your life and it's a real problem. It's mostly about what other people demand from you: your work, friends and family. You're under stress when you can't cope any more because events or circumstances have exceeded your ability to deal with them. In itself, stress is not a bad thing, but it can be harmful when stressful situations pile up instead of being dealt with one at a time.

Your work, friends and family all make demands on your time. Exercise and good food can help to reduce stress. They are positive steps you can take for yourself. You might think that exercise would add more stress to your life. After all, you'll have to make time in your day for it, won't you? This is true but you'll find that time can expand to accommodate exercise, just as the work any project requires will expand to fill (and overflow) the time you've got to do it. If you are fitter and eating well you will cope better with demands on your time, because your energy levels are better. You will cope better because you are more effective in your everyday life.

Exercising gives us a different perspective on other parts of our life as well. There's a kind of serenity in fitness. But it's pointless getting fit physically without trying to address your mental fitness too. After all, who wants to be able to do more press-ups than anyone else in the loony bin?

There are different types of stress, some big, some small, but it's all stress. Your body makes a physiological response to it by releasing adrenalin into your system, so your heart rate quickens, your metabolism speeds up and, in caveman terms, you're ready to fight the dinosaur. But the problem is you don't have a dinosaur to fight; you just have a gas bill. So what you end up with is chemicals in your body and an unbalanced feeling.

There is often an accumulation of stressful symptoms during one working day. For example, you drive to work in the rush hour. This makes you late for a meeting. The meeting goes badly and your best employee hands in his notice. You get home and your partner says 'What a day. I couldn't park at the shops.' You then explode because you've had the mother of all bad days and everyone else's life seems irrelevant compared to your own problems.

OK, deep down you know you are being unreasonable. The kids are important and your partner was probably out buying food for the family. This adds more stress, because now it's endangering your home life.

As the day goes on, you become more unbalanced. When you go to bed, you won't be able to sleep because your tiredness and inactivity are fighting each other.

Multiply this daily stress into a month, or a year, and it can build up into chronic stress. You could get some of the following: insomnia, bad skin conditions, high blood pressure, ulcers, tight muscle spasms, headaches and even cancer.

So how do you deal with it? The time-honoured solution is to have a drink. You come home, reach for the gin and flop on to the sofa and relax. But this doesn't work, because you don't feel relaxed the next morning, you just feel leaden. Alcohol is a depressant. It makes you feel horrible and sluggish next day.

Alcohol isn't harmful unless you drink too much of it. If it is linked to stress you'll find yourself drinking more and more to deal with the stress. And that reduces your ability to deal with the root problem.

You can also drink coffee to make you feel more alert and perk you up. But there is a cost. Coffee is a stimulant. It helps at first, but when you're on your tenth cup of the morning it can make you hyperactive and detract from your ability to cope. It makes your stomach feel bad and makes you feel awful.

It's much the same with cigarettes. They stimulate through the nicotine, but then you smoke 20 of them and negate the benefit. Nicotine makes you produce adrenalin artificially, and when you've got too much adrenalin in your system with nothing to do it makes you tired. More obviously, cigarettes ruin your health and that does nothing to reduce stress levels. Nicotine has almost exactly the same effect on you as the stress itself. Too much adrenalin is produced and it's got nowhere to go. This means you're lighting up a potential panic attack every time you have a cigarette.

You can take tranquillizers, sleeping pills, Prozac and all that other stuff to calm you down and to help you sleep at night. In theory, you should be more effective during the day. But these drugs can lead to psychological and physiological dependence.

The extreme solution is to go and live on a desert island, abandon your family and get rid of everything that causes you stress in your life. The painter Gaugin did this pretty successfully. So did the writer Ernest Hemingway, who was doing really well – right up to the point where he committed suicide.

A less extreme solution involves exercise and healthy eating. Stress-management experts regard exercise as an effective way of reducing stress symptoms. Doing something just for yourself releases tension. In addition, exercise is the dinosaur you can fight. The adrenalin coursing round your system is used for the purpose it was intended for. So when you hit a punch-bag you are slapping Jones from Accounts. You're working off frustration and aggression. That dissipates the adrenalin quicker. And it helps you to put things into perspective.

When I was learning to be a journalist I worked as a rock and roll truck-driver. Last year I was going through a sticky patch and got a phone call inviting me to go out on tour with Tina Turner for two weeks as a second driver. I went, but I was feeling homesick and miserable. Then one of the other truck-drivers started picking on me – 'OK, Mr Famous Journalist', that kind of thing. One night we were staying in a hotel in Warsaw and it got to the point where I really needed to smack him in the mouth. I went down to the gym and punched seven bells out of a punch-bag, swam 20 lengths and felt much better. I used the adrenalin that I had generated to hit the driver to bully the punch-bag instead. And, in so doing, I regained my perspective on the whole deal. What did I care? It wouldn't affect my life in general, just the next four days. On the way up to my room, I heard that after I left the driver had picked on someone else, who punched him in the mouth. They were both fired. So I got one up on him, and I used the experience in a positive way.

The other way to reduce stress is to eat better. Eating well is a symptom of being in control. If you hear someone saying they haven't got time to eat properly, they're not in control of their life. Stress is about being out of control. If you eat properly, your energy levels are much more balanced. If you go out and eat a big meal at lunchtime, when you come back to the office you're useless and the problems don't get solved because you're more ineffective.

The French sit down to lunch every day and they socialize and relax during a two-hour lunch break. That, combined with a healthy Mediterranean diet, means that they have one of the lowest incidences of heart disease in the world.

Deal with stress on a daily basis, if you can. This stops it becoming chronic. Fix things one at a time and achieve something every day. Hold on – we feel a car metaphor coming on. If your car is fixed every time it goes slightly wrong you get a load of small problems, but if you don't, the minor problems will begin to affect other parts of the machine. When you come to fix it, you may find it needs scrapping.

4
The Body

Your body is an incredible machine made up of different systems combining to make a (hopefully) harmonious whole. But you must look after it and keep it in good condition.

You don't need to understand the finer points of clutch design or the exact distance that a spark travels in your spark-plug to drive to the supermarket. But your relationship with your body is more personal, and it's important that you understand the rudimentary processes that keep you alive. Also when we ask you to do things, it will make some kind of sense to you and you will understand why.

Most people want their bodies to look good and to function perfectly for three-quarters of a century. Not only do they want this to happen with no maintenance, they also want to poison their systems with junk food, alcohol and cigarettes. But if you treat your body even half-way decently, it will do things for you that will amaze you and give you the added bonus of a terrific sense of well-being and happiness.

People who decide to get fitter or eat better immediately concentrate on the external appearance of the body. They want to get thin and fit *now*. Welcome to the modern world. But if you get liposuction or plastic surgery or buy miracle creams that will make the years drop off miraculously, you are addressing the signs of the problem, not the problem itself. The answer is nutrition and exercise. To solve the problems you have with your body, you need to aim for permanent well-being, not just a temporary fix.

We don't expect you to become a doctor, but, in that mess of muscles and chemical reactions that make up the body you've been using since birth, you were also given a fine brain. Please walk this way for Savill and Smedley's tour of the human body:

The vascular system

This is sometimes called the cardiovascular system. (Was ever a system so consistently abused by the human race in general?) It basically consists of the heart, blood, blood vessels, lymphatic vessels and lymph. But the star of this system is a large muscular pump known as the heart. This muscle continually pumps blood around the circulatory system, carrying oxygen and nutrients to the cells in your body.

The heart can pump at least 2.8 litres (5 pints) of blood around the body in one minute. It can pump even more when the body is being exerted during exercise or is under stress. During a 24-hour period, the adult human heart pumps approximately 36,000 litres (nearly 8000 gallons) of blood through 20,000 kilometres (12,400 miles) of blood vessels. That is amazingly efficient. I once had a pump that used to clear the bilges from an old boat I owned. It did 22.7 litres (five gallons) an hour. If you could invent a pump as small and efficient as the heart, you could afford to move to Hawaii and get Cindy Crawford to come round to your house and give you the live version of her exercise video.

The heart pumps blood to the lungs, where the blood cells pick up the oxygen that is needed by the body. It also takes the waste gases (carbon dioxide) and expels them into the lungs for exhalation via the mouth and/or nose. Again, a cool system. Imagine a car designed with a combined petrol filler-cap and exhaust system.

Blood vessels that come from the heart are called arteries. Once the blood leaves the heart and has picked up its oxygen from the lungs, and later nutrients from the digestion area, it sets off to deliver them around the body. The arteries branch out and become smaller. They are then called capillaries (after the Latin word for 'hair', because they are so thin and hair-like). The blood moves its nutrients and oxygen from the capillaries into the body tissue. At the same time the capillaries pick up the body's waste matter and carbon dioxide and take it back into the blood.

As the blood returns to the heart, it moves through venules (which are small veins) and then the veins themselves. These veins travel through waste-management organs such as the liver (most of the waste management components appear in mixed grills) and eventually return the blood to the heart, where the process begins again.

This miracle is provided free by nature. But, instead of marvelling that we don't need a degree to run such a complicated system, or a licence or tax, we spend most of our waking hours trying to stop it working. And we succeed remarkably well. Heart disease kills thousands of people every year and you are cordially invited to become one of them. Here's how:

- Eat fatty foods, go the extra sausage and eat lots of chicken khorma late at night. (You know how the waste-pipe under your sink gets clogged with grease all the time and you need to pour boiling water down it or take off the U-bend and put your fingers into unspeakable filth? Well, fatty food and no exercise produces the same effect, on your body, albeit slower. The boiling water is provided by exercise.)
- Don't exercise and get lots of stress.
- Eat badly and fur up your pipes. This isn't magic, this is physics.

Even when you're sitting on the sofa watching a quiz show your heart is working hard (even if your brain isn't). If you make your heart work harder than it needs to, you are inviting hypertension, arterial damage and injury to the heart.

The reason why a healthy heart works well is that each beat or pump of the heart produces a big wadge of blood to pump through the arteries and veins. A weak heart has to pump several times to do the same job. So, like the fat kid on the cross-country run, it works harder to achieve less. This is why business executives suffer from high blood pressure; they eat rich food, never exercise and have bucket-loads of stress. You're wondering what your blood pressure is, and, more importantly, what it should be. For now, all you can do is feel for a pulse inside your wrist. If you find one, go to the doctor and have your blood pressure taken. (If you haven't got a pulse, you're dead.) For those of you who are still reading, there is a table on page 26 that will tell you what your blood pressure ought to be.

The blood pressure readings are made up of two readings: the diastolic and the systolic. The diastolic is the reading when the heart is at the relaxed phase of the cycle and the systolic is when the heart is contracting. Blood pressure is expressed as a high number over a low number. So, if your blood pressure is 120/70, you're fine, and if it's 180/120 you're not well.

Optimum blood pressure readings for ages (adapted from World Health Organisation standard)

Age	20–24	25–29	30–34	35–39	40–44	45–49	50–54	55–59	60–64	65–69	70
MEN **systolic**											
max. blood pressure	142	142	145	148	151	158	170	177	184	188	197
min. blood pressure	114	114	113	112	113	114	118	123	128	128	133
diastolic											
max. blood pressure	88	88	91	94	95	97	103	104	107	106	106
min. blood pressure	62	62	63	63	67	69	71	72	72	72	72
WOMEN **systolic**											
max. blood pressure	134	137	139	144	152	166	175	178	188	196	202
min. blood pressure	108	107	109	110	112	114	119	122	128	136	140
diastolic											
max. blood pressure	84	85	87	91	93	100	101	104	106	106	107
min. blood pressure	60	61	63	65	67	68	71	72	74	76	75

Your blood pressure should be around the middle of the sections. My blood pressure before I started exercising was 159 (systolic) over 122 (diastolic). At the age of 42, this was not good at all. By the time I had exercised for three months it had dropped to 127 (systolic) over 75 (diastolic), pretty much where it is now, and that reading is fine for a 21-year-old. I tell you this not to boast (although I am a bit smug about it) but to show you that it can be done. If I can do it, you can. (Believe me: I weighed nearly 120 kilos [18 stone 10 lb], and that is not a pretty sight naked.) I also achieved it without a spectacular amount of effort.

The other benefit was that my heart-rate dropped from 80 BPM down to 66 BPM. Let's do the maths. On an average day my heart now beats 20,160 times less and that adds up to an astonishing

604,800 times a month. My heart is working far less to do the same job. I'll live to be a million. If you exercise, your heart works better, but it doesn't need to work as hard. It also helps to stop the build-up of cholesterol that clogs the arteries.

When you have a unhealthy life-style, stuff builds up in your arteries that you really don't want there. But when you exercise hard your blood acts like little Brillo pads and scrubs the arteries clean. This means that you get more blood rushing around, and it's cleaner and better, so you feel better too.

The respiratory system

The respiratory system supplies the body with oxygen and expels carbon dioxide from it. Put like that, it doesn't sound like that big a deal. But the average adult breathes roughly 13,650 litres (3000 gallons) of air a day. For the less technical among you, that's a lot. It constitutes not only the body's biggest daily intake, but the most vital. You can go without food for many days and without water for a few days, but even a few minutes without oxygen does horrible things to you.

During normal quiet breathing about 1.5 litres (2¹/2 pints) of air moves in and out of the lungs. This is known as tidal air. At the end of a normal breath, if you continue to breathe out you can force out another 1.5 litres (2¹/2 pints) of air.

If you never exercise, you don't expand your lungs and your breathing system just falls into disrepair. You need to exercise and get your heart rate up for at least five minutes before it does any real good. Your body will basically close down any part of the system not required by the management (that's you). When your breathing is working at peak efficiency, you don't notice it happening. It's only when your body's under load, running for the bus, that breathing becomes laboured and begins to be hard work.

Athletes reach the point where their breathing is still efficient even when they are exercising hard. That is why fit people (including you, when you've read this book) rarely appear out of breath.

Therefore, during our rebuilding of the magnificent you, we will have to concentrate on establishing the respiratory endurance you will need to exercise efficiently. This is because all physical exercise entails some of your muscles doing something, and muscles require oxygen to do anything at all. When muscles are operating, they heat up, and the oxygen delivered to them acts like a fuel, providing energy in intense bursts. As you become fitter, your lungs deliver oxygen more efficiently to your muscles and this means that more energy is available and performance improves. You become more efficient physically and, as your brain is also a user of oxygen, exercise may even improve your mental powers as well. (I know several people who are as fit as a fiddle yet couldn't string two words together – but it is a theory.)

People who exercise rarely are only too aware of the unpleasant feeling caused by being out of breath or not being able to catch their breath after walking upstairs or running for a bus. Aerobic exercise, even taken in moderation, will quickly turn you into the sort of person who is glad when the lift is broken, or who doesn't run for the bus but outruns it instead. (Well, not quite, but being fit enough to bend down to tie your shoelace rather than having to put your feet up on something is a relief in itself.)

Here's the good news. The lung bit and the heart bit not only work together in the body but when you start to behave they work better together as well. So you get a two-for-one deal.

So how do you know when it's all working better? When you have better stamina and your breathing improves when you do hard exercise.

Muscular skeletal system

The human body has 206 bones (count them if you want to). Bone itself is a living material made up of 25 per cent water, 30 per cent organic material and 45 per cent minerals, such as calcium and phosphate, which give the bones their rigidity.

These 206 bones make up the human skeleton, which is the framework of the human body. It has two functions: protection and locomotion. So the skull protects the brain, the ribcage protects the heart and lungs, and the spinal column stops the spinal cord from snapping.

It's the locomotion bit that concerns us here. It's a fact that if you regularly lift moderately heavy weights your skeletal health will improve. 'So what?' I hear you say. Well, in addition to the above functions, individual bones serve other purposes such as the attachment of tendons and muscles and the formation of red blood cells. What this means is that your current one-person crusade against nature will lead to nasty diseases that you probably can't even pronounce. Osteoporosis, for instance, is a withering deterioration of bone tissue which softens and weakens the bones. Extensive research shows that regular exercise, such as working with weights, can prevent this condition.

We all have over 600 muscles, even weedy blokes. Some of them work on orders from the brain via the central nervous system and some just do their own thing. The ones that take no crap from the management are mostly involved in the beating of the heart, breathing and digestion. For obvious reasons, these have their own union.

The basic shape we are is determined not only by the size of our bones, but also by the shape of our skeletal voluntary muscles. These nearly always work in co-ordinated groups so that the contraction of one results in the stretching of another. Because skeletal muscles are attached to two or more bones, when one contracts the bones attached to it move. The skeletal system relies on muscles to move it and to make it stand up. If you don't exercise, you get back or hip problems or bad knees. People in offices often spend their time sitting badly and then they get physical problems, because their bad posture has weakened their muscles.

But not us – we are going to exercise and look after our health. We are going to make fitness a cornerstone of the new us. Muscles will adapt to achieve what they are asked to do. So if your main mission in life is to eat hamburgers, your jaws will end up wonderfully strong, but the rest of you will go to hell in a handcart. If you compare the muscle mass of a lumberjack with that of Colin from accounts, you'll see what we mean.

When you start to exercise your muscles by doing weight-lifting or running, for example, you alert them to the fact that you're going to be asking something different of them. As you get them to move within their natural range of motion with enough intensity, the muscle cells break down. But the good news is that they rebuild themselves stronger and become more efficient, given good nutrition.

What we want to teach you is the premise that not only you can make yourself stronger (able to lift that weight, for example), but you will soon gain muscular endurance (lift the weight a number of times). You need to concentrate on both of these aspects to gain proper fitness. The more efficient muscle will look good on the beach as well!

Muscles need energy just to exist. So a good muscle mass is busy consuming calories even when it's not doing anything, and this stops calories building up fat deposits. The opposite side of this coin is that you have to eat healthily to maintain the muscle mass, or it will wither away.

The digestive system

Your digestive system plays an important part in maintaining your energy levels. During the digestive process, the large bits of protein, carbohydrates and fat you eat in a meal are broken down into simpler substances your body can absorb and use for fuel.

The human digestive system is made up of the following: the mouth, the oesophagus (or gullet), the stomach, the small intestine, the large intestine and the anus. Other starring roles in this process go to the glandular organs, which include the salivary glands, the liver, the gall bladder and the pancreas.

Let's follow that meal down, shall we? First it's ground up in the mouth and saliva is added via glands in the cheeks and tongue. This isn't where the really big action happens on the digestive front. The mouth is home to a little splitting enzyme called amylase.

As the food hits the stomach, it mixes with digestive juices and is churned by the muscular walls of the stomach. This mixture is called chyme and, depending on the kind of food it is, it stays as a guest of the stomach for about three to five hours. It then goes off down to the small intestine. At this point more enzymes are mixed with it to break it down into its component parts so it can be absorbed into the bloodstream. In the small intestine, a membrane takes out the fat and sugar and pushes them into the bloodstream. Most of the goodness is taken out of the meal by the small intestine.

The rest of the material, including undigested fibres, unabsorbed food components and dead cells, is moved on into the large intestine with wavelike contractions of the intestine called peristalsis.

Note: Chew your food much more thoroughly. If you chew your food well, it makes it taste better and it's easier to digest. Also, if you spend longer eating, you will (paradoxically) eat less. Don't believe me? Watch any fat person eating. In the case of most fatties, eating is the fastest thing they ever do.

Even more happens here. Water and salt are extracted and then it's chucked down to the colon, where it's all but done.

The metabolism

Your metabolism governs the rate at which you burn the calories contained in your food. This rate obviously varies from person to person. It is the part of us we most often blame for making us fat. 'It's not my fault I've got a slow metabolism.' If you filled it up with crap fuel, you'd have a slow Ferrari. Your base metabolism is defined as the number of calories your body will burn in a day if you do nothing at all. Anything you do, even watching telly, will boost your calorie need. If you exercise, your calorie requirement will go up even more.

Whatever your metabolic rate is, aerobic exercise will speed it up for about six hours afterwards. It's a bit like a moving car; if you switch the engine off, it will take a while to stop. If you increase the size of your muscles, they in turn will use up even more calories and this speeds up your metabolism as well. So does this mean you can eat mountains of bacon sandwiches and be thin as a whip? Well, no, but if you're exercising a lot, you can relax a bit.

Your metabolic rate is created by your eating habits, genetic inheritance and daily exercise. You can't change the genetic bit, you're stuck with that, but you can alter the other factors so that it becomes less important. As we go through the book, we are going to kick ass on the metabolic front (!).

Blood sugar levels

Your body doesn't ask much. What it needs is energy (in the form of glucose), delivered to your muscles at a consistent and methodical rate as long as it's expending it normally. In this way, the energy that it gets it uses. It's simple, economical and has worked for thousands of years. Your body likes this cycle, whereby it picks up energy in a steady stream. But there's a problem: you.

You like to mess about with the order of things. You go on diets, and the energy isn't delivered in sufficient quantity. Then you get low blood sugar, which is called hypoglycaemia. Or you go on a curry-and-lager blow-out and deliver the Hiroshima protein bomb to your system – yes, you guessed it, high blood sugar or hyperglycaemia. Either way you go, it's called blood sugar imbalance.

When energy levels get low, the body registers that it has a problem and calls for instant energy fixes. This is when you get the munchies. The sugary stuff you eat is quickly digested and enters the bloodstream at speed. Then your blood sugar levels hit the roof. Your body protects itself from this energy surge by producing a large dose of insulin. The insulin curbs the excess energy, but does it in such a way that it over-compensates and reduces the blood sugar to a level below what your body is comfortable with. In other words, you end up with low blood sugar and the whole cycle starts again. So the big lump of chocolate you eat when you feel crappy is just a temporary fix at best, though quite a tasty one.

If you overeat at mealtimes, the same thing happens, but at a different point in the cycle. When you take in a load of high-energy food at lunch, your blood sugar levels skyrocket. Your pancreas releases its large dose of insulin and your blood sugar levels crash. Then your body sends out for the energy cavalry. You suddenly feel the need for a sugar bomb-out and you're back where you were before. Richard calls this 'the negative insulin cycle'.

Dieting slows down your metabolism. When you diet, you aim to keep your blood sugar levels consistently low, which is why you always crave sweet food, and why the whole concept is doomed to failure. People nearly always crash their diets with a sweet binge for this reason.

Us clever types will ensure that we eat little and often so our blood sugar levels will cease their roller-coaster ride and we will always have the energy we need.

The set point

Weight loss supposedly depends on reducing your calorie intake and exercising more, so that you burn more calories than you eat. If you go on long enough, you'll look like Kate Moss on a very thin day. (Well, not quite.) But because your body has an optimum set point, where it naturally feels happy, this can disrupt the 'calorie in, calorie out' equation to which a lot of people adhere.

I fell from over 110 kilos (18 stone) to 92 kilos (14½ stone), but the weight I can maintain really easily is 95 kilos (15 stone). I like weighing 92 kilos, but my wife thinks I look gaunt, so it seems that my body's set point is 95 kilos. That's where I feel right, and alarm bells ring if I go more than a few grams over this weight. It's the outer limit for my health and happiness in weight terms.

You have to fix realistic goals for your set point. I'm 1.5 metres (6 foot 5 inches) tall, and I'm never going to weigh as little as 50 kilos (8 stone), no matter how hard I try. We also want you to change permanently, so it's worth taking a while to reach your set point. If you lose loads of weight in a hurry, you are fairly likely to regain some – or all – of the weight you lost.

If you lose weight at a reasonable rate, eat right and exercise all the way down the scales, you are selling your body the idea of a new you slowly, and it is more likely to respond favourably. The unfortunate fact is that the longer your body sits at a certain weight, the harder it is for this to change dramatically.

Now you know you have a set point, but how do you find out what it is? The following method (calculated in Imperial measures) will give you an approximate idea of what you should weigh, so you have a goal figure.

- A man should weigh 106 pounds for the first five feet of his height. Add 6 pounds for each inch of height, plus or minus 10 per cent (depending on frame size).

    For example, I'm 6 foot 5 inches tall. The calculation would work out like this:

$$106 \text{ lb} + (17 \text{ inches} \times 6 \text{ lb}) = 208 \text{ lb}$$

This is a weight of 14 stone 12 pounds, which is almost exactly right for me.

- For women, the calculation is based on a weight of 100 pounds for the first five feet, adding 5 pounds per inch after that height.

The real test is to stand in front of the mirror and look at yourself with a harsh eye. Bend forward a bit, don't breathe in. You almost certainly know what your ideal weight is, either instinctively, or because you've been at that weight at some stage in your life.

5
Nutrition

Just after the Romanian revolution, I was part of an orphanage expedition that took a sixty-foot truck into mountains which had never been visited by western Europeans. We entered a country that was short of everything in a truck full of diesel, with the sure knowledge that we didn't have enough fuel to get out again. In the end we found that we were able to buy supplies from tractors parked by the side of the road. The cost per litre was insanely cheap but the fuel was watered down to such an extent that we could only buy half a tankful at a time in the hope that the better stuff would mix with the rubbish and get the truck home. But that was in an emergency. Imagine pulling into a garage on a major motorway in Europe to buy fuel that you know contains elements which are harmful to your engine. Unthinkable, huh?

Every day of our lives we make that same choice when it comes to our own fuel, by eating bad food – and we think nothing of it. Like all machines, our bodies operate on the fuel we give them. The better the fuel, the better the performance we can expect. Unfortunately, we have a tendency to reach for junk food. This results in poor performance, so we feel terrible.

If you try to get fit without bothering about nutrition, you're wasting your time. And if you don't make it you're not helping our book sales either. It's not difficult to construct a detailed nutrition plan for someone. They don't work, though. In fact, these plans become increasingly useless in direct proportion to how complicated they are. Let's face it, we're blokes. To us a pulse isn't something we associate with food, it's something we search for in the morning to find out if we have survived the night before.

Counting calories and weighing food the whole time is just too much trouble and, to be honest, this side of nutrition isn't that critical, as long as the overall picture is right. Also, you haven't got time, because you've got a life, haven't you? (Well, don't worry, you will have when we've made you thin and healthy. It worked for me – I'm getting turned down by much better-looking and younger women now.)

Calculating calories can make you obsessive about eating, too. And it restricts your social life because you're so busy thinking about those little calories that you become pain in the ass.

You can follow set menus that take you through 30-day eating plans. The problem with them is that they're not designed for you as an individual. They take no account of the fact that you will find yourself tired and needing food at inconvenient times. In addition, you are putting yourself in the control of someone you've never met. (Yeah, yeah, I know, but it's different with us. We want your friends to buy the book too, so we have your best interests at heart.)

So what's our plan? Well, we're blokes and we like machines. If we find out how food works in the same way as we find out how our VCR works, we will carry the knowledge with us. These food groups are components which we use to make ourselves healthy (and if we are lucky, we can achieve this without having too many bits left over at the end).

We'll look at the six basic food types, which are:

- carbohydrates
- proteins
- fats
- vitamins
- minerals
- water.

We'll learn what they do and how our body reacts to them, which food groups turbo-charge us and which are just go-faster stripes. Once we understand the six basic food types we can work out for ourselves what we need to drive our body so we can get fit and look good.

Carbohydrates contain carbon and water and are the body's main source of energy. Most carbohydrates also include fibre-bulky plant materials. These aid digestion and waste management. They also reduce cholesterol. You can see why we need them. If we eat too much carbohydrate and don't exercise, our engine's running fast, but it's not in gear. So it becomes fat.

Proteins form the structural framework of living cells. Every piece of our bodies, including our skin, brain, lungs, heart, bowel muscle, and even our teeth has some kind of protein as its basic material.

Fats, also called lipids, give you energy and insulation. The body also uses small amounts of fat to repair and enlarge some tissue.

Vitamins are the good guys. These are complex chemicals that the body keeps for sustenance and operations. They act as catalysts and are essential to the overall workings of the body. Only small amounts are needed.

Minerals are vital to maintaining physiological processes. One more machine analogy – they are the oil of the body.

Water, which is not actually a food group, is included because of its importance to our plan. Water increases blood volume, transports nutrients and makes up about two-thirds of muscular tissue. It also eliminates waste and regulates body temperature. We lose about 2.3 litres (4 pints) of water a day via bodily functions like sweating, breathing and excreting. So you've got to drink at least six or seven glasses of water a day to maintain a proper level of hydration. (And when we say water we mean water, not the sort you buy in pints that has been mixed with hops and stuff.)

Calorie content of the six basic food types

carbohydrates and protein	4 calories per gram
fats	9 calories per gram
vitamins, minerals and water	0 calories per gram

So how much do I need of these nutrients?

Vitamins and mineral supplements are covered properly if your carbohydrate and fat intake is eaten in the right amounts and comes from nutritious fresh food. The really important point is to make sure that your carbohydrate, protein and fat intake are balanced. The American food guide pyramid system illustrated below is a great help here. It is easy to use and simplifies the whole quantity/calorie/food-weight business.

The food guide pyramid, showing recommended daily servings from the different food groups

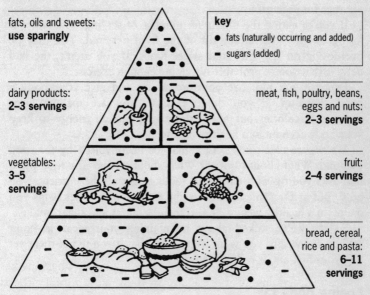

fats, oils and sweets:
use sparingly

key
● fats (naturally occurring and added)
▬ sugars (added)

dairy products:
2–3 servings

meat, fish, poultry, beans, eggs and nuts:
2–3 servings

vegetables:
3–5 servings

fruit:
2–4 servings

bread, cereal, rice and pasta:
6–11 servings

(Source: US Department of Agriculture)

You will immediately see that the recommended servings are not set out dogmatically, which means that you don't have to split the atom just to eat a meal. The number of servings is stated as a window, with a minimum and maximum for each group. If you've got a big frame, you'll probably eat around the top of the servings suggestions. If you're medium build, graze in the middle. If you're small-framed, you should be aiming towards the bottom of the serving suggestions. Base your frame size on what your weight should be, not what it is now. Remember the calculation in the last chapter and use it.

The pyramid system allows you to personalize your intake and gives you helpful guidelines to follow. Your intake is not set in stone and you need to practise a degree of micro-management on a daily basis. By making small adjustments to your consumption of calories, you'll soon learn what works for your metabolism.

Believe me, if you are doing this right you will almost certainly lose weight. To achieve the weight loss you want, stay within the guidelines. If you don't lose weight even though you really are staying within them, you may need to decrease the number of servings for each group.

If you're eating the minimum number of servings and still not losing weight, look at the tip of the food pyramid. You may be overdosing on the fatty and sweet foods. If you aren't, the bad news is that you're probably not doing enough exercise.

Exercise will mobilize your stored fat and give your body a good shake-up. If you don't exercise, you are making large deposits of calories but not withdrawing enough energy to keep your body account at a healthy balance.

We realize that some people may be unconvinced by the food pyramid. What about calories? What about grams? The food pyramid asks you to eat a variety of foods to get all the nutrients you need. But at the same time the right amount of calories helps you maintain a healthy weight. It also focuses on fat and sugar intake.

So far we've talked about maintaining your ideal set-point weight, the weight you want to be. But what if you're not there yet and your first aim is to lose body fat?

Losing body fat

Below is a chart that will give you a starting-point to lose body fat.

Weight-loss mode serving suggestions

Group	Servings per day	Small frame		Medium frame		Large frame	
		Men	Women	Men	Women	Men	Women
fats, oils, sweets	M*	M	M	M	M	M	M
dairy products	2–3	2.5	2.0	2.5	2.5	3.0	2.5
meat, fish, poultry, beans, eggs, nuts	2–3	2.5	2.0	2.5	2.5	3.0	2.5
vegetables	3–5	3.5	3.0	4.0	3.5	4.5	4.0
fruits	2–3	2.0	2.0	2.5	2.5	3.0	3.0
breads, cereals, rice and pasta	6–11	7.0	6.0	8.0	7.0	9.0	8.0
Approximate calories per day		1400–1600		1600–1800		1800–2000	

* minimize (M)

I followed the large frame serving guide and almost never felt hungry. The servings assume that you are doing some of the exercises that we tell you about later. The good news is that if you exercise a lot you can increase the amount in the bread, cereals, rice and pasta group right from the start. If you suddenly find that you're Linford Christie and you like exercise more than you thought, you need to increase your intake of all the food groups. Remember to increase them gradually to find your own level. Give yourself a little leeway.

What constitutes a serving?

In this section we set out recommended serving suggestions within the context of the food groupings on the pyramid. Most are given by weight or using visualization methods (in plain language, what the serving looks like). Once you know that an 85-gram (3-ounce) piece of meat or fish is about the same size as a deck of cards, for example, you just make sure that you eat that much next time.

The bread, cereal, rice and pasta group

This is an important group. You need six to eleven servings of this stuff a day.

One serving equals:

- one average slice of bread
- half a cup of cooked cereal, rice, pasta, grains or diced potatoes
- three tablespoons of breakfast cereal (not the sugary kind)
- one small bagel.

The fruit group

Eat two to four servings of fruit a day. This group includes fresh fruit, but can as a back-up include canned, juiced or dried fruit. Dried or canned fruit should be limited because of their raised sugar and reduced vitamin content. What you want is nice, natural, organic fruit.

One serving equals:

- one cup of strawberries or raspberries, blackberries or logan-berries
- one medium-sized apple, orange, pear, peach, grapefruit or apricot
- one wineglassful of fruit juice
- half a cup of cooked or canned fruit
- one small banana
- a cupful of grapes.

The vegetable group

Eat three to five servings of these trusty little devils each day. As you know, these are the good guys.

The vegetable group includes fresh, frozen or canned vegetables. Fresh vegetables are best, preferably organic, and eaten raw they are better still. Raw vegetables maximize your intake of vitamins, minerals and fibre. Frozen vegetables are OK. Canned ones should really be used only as a back-up.

One serving of vegetables equals, for instance:

- half a cup of raw or cooked broccoli, corn, Brussels sprouts, green beans, squash or other vegetables of that ilk
- three-quarters of a cup of tomatoes or onion
- one cup of cooked leafy vegetables
- half a cup of peas, carrots or beetroot
- a small bowl of mixed salad.

Meat, fish, poultry, dry beans, eggs and nuts

What this lot does is to supply high-quality protein. This can be a dangerous group. You can make merry with the vegetables, but this group has to be treated with respect. (That is, if you feel that you can treat nuts with respect!)

A lot of the foods in this group contain fat and this can be a problem if not controlled. However, chosen carefully, fats can be kept within the normal bounds for health and well-being. Nuts especially contain loads of calories and should be avoided, except at Christmas. And they are salty, which makes you want to drink more. (OK, you've heard that peanuts are good for your sex life, but if you eat too many, you won't have a sex life.)

One serving from this group would be:

- 85 grams (3 ounces) of cooked beef or chicken without the skin (a serving is about the size of a deck of cards).
- one cup of cooked beans (black-eyed, red, etc.)
- 85 grams (3 ounces) of cooked fish (again, the same size as a deck of cards)
- one egg – reduce fat and cholesterol by eating only the white of the egg.

The milk, yoghurt and cheese group (dairy products)

Two to three servings each day are your ration from this group. If you choose wisely, your fat intake will not be a problem. If you want to drink milk, make it the skimmed kind, especially when you're in the weight-loss bit of the programme.

Eat yoghurt and cheese, but buy the low-fat sort. Keep away from hard cheese; it is generally much higher in saturated fat than the softer kinds, like cottage cheese or cheese spreads.

A serving in this group equals:

- one cup of milk
- a small carton of yoghurt
- 28 grams (1 ounce) of hard cheese
- 56 grams (2 ounces) of processed cheese
- two cups of cottage cheese.

The fats, oils and sweets group

These are the dangerous brothers. It's important to get this group right, for weight loss and general health, because it is usually the one that causes weight gain.

Let's start with fats. Because fat is naturally present in a lot of the other food groups, it is not something you should add to food or your frying-pan. Dairy, fish and meat products are generally quite high in fat, so take care to use the lower-fat varieties. As a guide, if you want to lose weight, eat 30 to 40 grams a day, and no more than 60 grams a day when maintaining your correct weight. If you buy ready-made foods, try to choose meals that contain roughly 5 grams of fat per 100 grams of the product.

Cut out or cut down on cakes, sweets, pies and desserts. They generally provide too much energy to use under normal circumstances and may cause the negative insulin cycle. As we said earlier, you should avoid this situation.

All this gives a rough framework to plan your eating in terms of food groups and the servings you need on a daily basis. Everyone is different, so serving quantities will vary.

Proportional balance of food groups

Nutritionists recommend that we should eat our food groups in the following proportions:

- 65 per cent of calories from carbohydrates
- 15 per cent of calories from proteins
- 20 per cent of calories from fats.

But the problem is that it's hard to figure out what you are eating proportionally. Some foods contain carbohydrates, protein and fat. Milk, for example, contains all three. So how do you work out your calculations? Well, you can rely on the food pyramid guide, because it approximates the servings in the right proportions.

It's never going to be 100 per cent accurate, but it doesn't need to be. We are working to wider tolerances here, and if you miss by a bit it's not the end of the world. It is certainly a realistic way of eating in the right proportions without hiring a nutritionist to follow you around.

Servings turned into meals

Some of the serving suggestions sound quite a lot, don't they? Eleven servings of carbohydrates sounds like a sack of spuds! But here's how the servings relate to real-life meal portions:

Bread, cereal, rice and pasta group (6–11 servings)

	Serving size	Portion at meal	Number of servings
cereal	3 tbsp	6–9 tbsp	2–3
bread	1 slice	2 slices	2
bagel	small	one big	2
pasta	half a cup, cooked	2–3 cups	4–6
rice	half a cup, cooked	1–2 cups	2–4

Six to eleven servings are only two to four servings per meal or the equivalent of about 150 to 300 calories.

The fruit group (2–4 servings)

	Serving size	Portion at meal	Number of servings
apple juice	1 wineglass	2 glasses	2
apple	1 medium	1 large	2
banana	1 small	1 large	2
canned fruit	half a cup	1 cup	2

The vegetable group (2–4 servings)

	Serving size	Portion at meal	Number of servings
broccoli	1 small stalk	2 big stalks	3–4
spinach	1 cup	275 g (10 oz)	3
salad bar	small bowl	big bowl	2–3
spaghetti sauce	half a cup	1 cup	2

Meat, fish, poultry, beans, eggs and nuts (2–3 servings)

	Serving size	Portion at meal	Number of servings
tuna	half a 175-g (6-oz) can	1 whole can	2
chicken breast	85 g (3 oz)	175 g (6 oz)	2
peanut butter	2 tbsp	2–4 tbsp	1–2
lentil soup	1 cup	1 bowl	2
kidney beans	half a cup	1 cup	2

Dairy products (2–3 servings)

	Serving size	Portion at meal	Number of servings
milk (low fat)	1 cup	1½ cups	1.5
yoghurt (low fat)	1 pot	2 pots per day	2
cheese	25 g (1 oz)	50 g (2 oz)	2
cottage cheese	1 cup	3 cups	3

So, how are you doing?

By now you should be getting the idea that food must be eaten in the right proportions and the correct servings for your individual needs. But there's more we need to tell you about the best choice of foods within each main group for you to eat every day. Some foods are better than others because of their fat, sugar, vitamin or mineral content, their effect on your blood sugar levels, or just the way they make you feel.

I'd like to lighten things up a bit here. You don't need to totally exclude your favourite fattening food. The chances are that if you are following our plan you will crave less anyway.

Try to remember that no one food makes for complete nutrition. So your plan to go on to 2000 calories a day entirely fuelled by bottled beer is a crap one. I know, I tried it for 42 years.

We're trying to steer you into a state where you choose the better track naturally and then these food choices become easier. Statistically, at least one person's life will be changed for ever by this book. Let's make it you, shall we?

6
Carbohydrates

Carbohydrates are found in the pyramid food groups in the following categories:

- dairy products
- vegetables
- grains, cereals, rice, pasta, bread
- beans and nuts in the high-protein group.

Not all foods in these groups are heavily made up from carbohydrates, but they do contain them in varying proportions.

Carbohydrates used to be split into two groups. In one was the starchy, complex carbohydrate that contains long chains of sugar molecules joined together like beads on a string. These are technically termed polysaccharides. The other sort was the simple or sugary carbohydrate which consists of monosaccharides or disaccharides.

Whether the carbohydrate you eat starts life as the starchy, complex type or the simple sugary type, your body breaks it down into glucose and then uses it as fuel, carried to your cells by your blood.

The traditional way of classifying carbohydrates by their chemical structure, with no regard to the effect they have on the body, is now outdated. It was widely believed that complex carbohydrates, or starches like rice or potatoes, were slowly digested and absorbed, so they would only cause a small rise in blood sugar levels. On the other hand, simple carbohydrates were assumed to be digested and absorbed quickly. They would then produce a large and rapid increase in blood sugar.

In literal terms, these assumptions were wrong. We now think in terms of quick- and slow-release carbohydrates. The reason it is important to know which ones are quick- or slow-release concerns their effect on your blood sugar levels. If you always eat carbohydrates that release energy quickly your blood sugar levels will rise and cause excessive insulin release. In addition to causing low blood sugar, excessive amounts of insulin in your system will prevent your stored body fat being easily released as a source of energy. This will clearly not help in reducing your body fat levels and could actually cause them to rise.

The glycaemic index (GI)

High, moderate and low GI carbohydrates

This index is a chart, formulated by nutritionists and scientists, of common carbohydrate foods that are measured against the blood sugar or glycaemic response of glucose. Glucose's response is quantified as 100 on the scale and the other foods are measured against it. The lower the figure of a food, the slower it releases its energy into the bloodstream. Obviously, the higher the figure, the faster. Beer, for instance, has a GI or glycaemic value of 110. Cherries are in the low 20's. By understanding which types of foods are likely to be high or low we can make considered choices to our advantage.

What determines GI values?

Different factors will affect the glycaemic, or GI, value of a carbohydrate. Fibre, for example, slows down the access of digestive enzymes to the starch in our intestines, so fibre-rich carbohydrates are a good idea. The less a fibre is processed, and left in its natural state with its starch, the better. Intact whole-wheat grains are low GI. Once made into fine flour, their GI value rises.

Processing is another factor. When you mill grains into flour, juice fruits or reconstitute cereals, you heighten their GI values because they become easier and quicker for your body to digest. So choose breads high in whole-grains, and eat the whole fruit, not its juice. Try to eat unprocessed cereals like porridge or low-sugar muesli, not cornflakes or Rice Krispies, which are reconstituted.

Cooking affects GI values as well. Some starch granules swell up or, in some cases, burst when cooked. This leads to easier digestive-enzyme access and raises GI levels. The starch in potatoes baked for long periods swells up more than when they are boiled. This is why baked potatoes have a higher GI value than boiled potatoes, which don't swell so much. When cooked, the starch in some rice bursts and makes it sticky. This type of rice has the highest GI. Rice that forms separate pieces when cooked is generally lower GI for this reason.

Pasta is low to moderate GI because the durum wheat used is very hard in granule form and does not swell or burst so much.

Fat slows down the speed at which you digest carbohydrates. For instance, crisps are lower GI than boiled potatoes. But don't base your carbohydrate choices on items that are low GI because of the fat. Crisps are low GI, but they are low GI because of the fat, which you should be avoiding. (There's more about this on page 50.)

The amount you eat of a carbohydrate won't affect its GI value, but if you eat too much of even a low GI carbohydrate, it will affect your blood sugar level badly. So you should limit the amount of higher GI carbohydrates that you eat. Make sure that your food pyramid serving suggestion numbers are the moderate-to-low GI types.

Are we saying that high GI foods should be left out of an eating programme? No, we're not, but they do need to be treated with respect. High GI carbohydrates are best eaten after exercise. If you have to eat them, perhaps at a friend's house for dinner, eat them in small quantities. Low to moderate GI foods should be eaten before exercise, because they provide substantial endurance energy and should therefore form the main part of your everyday carbohydrate intake.

To simplify high, low and medium GI, there follows quite a comprehensive list of everyday foods. We have divided them like this:

- High GI foods – within the 60–100 bracket
- Moderate GI foods – within the 40–60 bracket
- Low GI foods – any carbohydrate below 40.

The GI content of some of the foods listed is based on an average, and some GI ratings will vary depending on who is eating them. Remember also that high fat content in a carbohydrate cushions the sugar release, so although they are desirable from their low GI value, their fat content means they should be avoided.

High GI

glucose	100	rice pasta	92
French baguette	95	rice (instant 6-minute kind)	91
Lucozade drink	95	rice (waxy, sticky kind)	88
corn muffin	95	baked potato	85
parsnips	95	cornflakes	84

pretzel snack	83	white bread	69
Rice Krispies	82	canned drink	68
rice cakes	82	Mars bar	68
tapioca pudding	81	Kellogg's Sustain	68
puffed crispbread	81	cornflour	68
broad beans	79	gnocchi pasta	68
Coco pops	77	Nutrigrain cereal	66
doughnut	76	grapenuts	66
waffles	76	orange cordial	66
pumpkin	75	fresh pineapple	66
corn bread	75	green pea soup	66
French fries	75	barley flour bread	66
Cheerios cereal	74	couscous	65
bread stuffing	74	rye flour bread	65
Graham crackers	74	table sugar	65
honey	73	melon	65
swede	72	beetroot	64
corn chips	72	raisins	64
watermelon	72	shortbread biscuits	64
bagel (white)	72	porridge	61
carrots	71	hamburger bun	61
Melba toast	70	ice cream (full fat)	61
Shredded Wheat	69	muesli bars	61
wholemeal bread	69		

Moderate GI

bran muffin	60	pumpernickel flour bread	50
pizza base	60	low-fat ice cream	50
split pea soup	60	linguini pasta	49
pawpaw	60	grapefruit juice	48
Bran Buds cereal	58	green peas	48
chappati (white flour)	57	bulgar wheat	48
kiwi fruit	57	baked beans	48
orange juice	57	white parboiled rice	47
boiled potatoes	56	oat bran bread	47
white long-grain rice	56	grapes	47
sultanas	56	instant noodles	47
muesli	56	pineapple juice	46
fruit cocktail (in syrup)	55	barley kernel bread	46
mango	55	capellini pasta	45
brown rice	55	macaroni	45
popcorn	55	lentil soup	44
sweetcorn	55	oranges	44
Special K	54	50% kibbled wheat-grain bread	43
bulgar flour bread	52	custard	43
banana (overripe)	52	All Bran	42
sultana bran cereal	52	peaches	42
peaches in light syrup	52	spaghetti (durum wheat)	41
yam	51	apple juice (unsweetened)	41

Low GI

barley kernel bread	40	butter beans	31
pasta – ravioli (with meat)	39	green beans	30
plums	39	dried beans	29
tomato soup	38	lentils	29
pasta (wholemeal)	37	whole milk	27
apples	36	grapefruit juice	25
pears	36	fructose	23
vermicelli pasta	35	dried peas	22
chocolate milk	34	cherries	22
Power Bar	30–35	rice bran cereal	19
low-fat yoghurt	33	soya beans	15
chick-peas	33	peanuts	14
fettuccini pasta	32	low-fat yoghurt with artificial	
skimmed milk	32	sweetener	14
split peas	32	apricots	7
dried apricots	31		

(High, moderate and low GI foods is adapted from *The GI Factor* by Professor Jennie Brand Miller, Kaye Foster Powell and Dr Stephen Colagiuri [Hodder & Stoughton, 1996])

At the beginning, when you're trying to lose weight, or if you've been naughty and you're trying to lose weight again, the following advice may help.

Fruit

Fruits that have stones are usually low GI, so try to eat these regularly. We're talking plums, apricots, cherries and the like.

Eat apples in preference to oranges as a snack, as they have a lower GI value.

Use high GI fruit at the end of a long work-out when your blood sugar is low and you need the boost.

When you want fruit, eat fruit. Fruit juice has a higher GI value than the fruit it comes from. But if you want to drink juice, drink apple juice rather than orange juice, because it's lower GI. Stay away from high GI juices like pineapple.

Vegetables and legumes

Try to make the lower value GI vegetables your mainstay. But go ahead and party with the higher ones occasionally.

Reduce your potato intake at most of your meals. Potatoes are fattening, as are most root vegetables, such as swede and parsnips – but you know that already, don't you?

Bean salad of any description is a good alternative. Although high in carbohydrate, beans generally have half the GI rating of the spud.

Whole-wheat pasta such as vermicelli, fettuccini or spaghetti is another good alternative, unless it's covered with oily sauces.

Leafy vegetables are very low in the GI department and you are invited to chomp on millions of them to your heart's content.

Carrots are very high on the GI. The message here is, eat them – they're great in vitamin contents and minerals – but don't overdose on them. Have a couple of raw carrots as a snack, especially after a work-out.

Bread

All breads are not created equal. What you need to eat are the lower GI types because they are better for you. Find out which kind of the lower GI ones you like the best and buy those. Simple, huh?

French baguettes have a very high reading and so are best avoided.

The more whole-grain breads have more vitamins and minerals, the best of all being pumpernickel. And actually it doesn't taste that bad. Eventually.

Pasta

Pasta is an important source of carbohydrate energy. The whole-meal variety has the benefit of fibre, which is good for you although some find it unpalatable. Try using a mixture of white and brown durum flour when making pasta for that killer seduction meal.

Pasta gets a bad press, but more often than not it's the sauce that's to blame. The durum wheat grain is extremely hard and breaks cleanly into distinct small pieces. This makes it difficult for you to digest and so it has low GI. Try not to eat pasta more than twice a week and use low-fat sauces.

If you overeat any food you get fat, so make sure that the portions you eat are within the pyramid serving suggestions. You have to be especially vigilant with pasta; it's easy to shovel in the stuff without thinking.

Cereals

Breakfast sets you up for the day. By eating a low GI cereal with skimmed milk, you reduce your chances of suffering the low blood sugar blues in the middle of the morning. And if you do get them, you will start wanting to eat bad, instant-energy foods like sweets and sausage rolls.

Choose cereals that have low GI and haven't been messed about with too much. All Bran and muesli are good options here. But don't be too heavy-handed with the portions, and remember to use skimmed milk.

Rice

Rice generally has a high GI value and some types have very high ones. Basmati rice is the lower GI type of rice. Wild rice is a good option. Stay away from the sticky type of rice.

Try keeping rice a low-fat option by not smothering it in oil. Cook it in fresh stocks and use plenty of herbs.

Beans

Beans are a very good source of carbohydrate. They have a low fat content, a low GI and are high in vitamin and mineral content. So we recommend that you eat them on a regular basis.

GI values and weight control

If you eat lower GI type carbohydrates on a regular basis you will stop the see-saw effect of high blood sugar levels and therefore minimize surplus energy being stored as body fat. There will be times when your blood sugar levels are low, such as after exercising, and you will need to eat high GI carbohydrates, like bananas or oranges, or starchy type foods such as a bagel. In that instance high GI intake is actually helpful.

Even though potatoes, bread and rice are high GI you can still eat them, but it is better to restrict their intake to no more than three servings at any one meal. So if you're eating pizza, for example, avoid the garlic bread.

The effect of low GI food at one meal carries over to the next meal and reduces the glycaemic value of that meal too. Even if you eat a low GI meal for dinner, the effect carries over to breakfast the next morning. So the aim is to eat two low GI meals a day and in the absence of a work-out make sure your snacks are low GI, too.

Other important points about carbohydrates

The question is, 'Do carbohydrates make you fat?' For many years people believed that sugar and starchy foods like pasta, rice and potatoes were the main culprits in making people obese.

So many diets just restrict the intake of carbohydrates. And you can lose weight that way. But most of the weight loss in these programmes is due to losing fluid, not body fat. This type of diet depletes your glycogen stores, the fuel your body makes by breaking down carbohydrates. As a result, you become tired and listless.

Actually, most fatties aren't fat because of the carbohydrates they eat, but because of the oils and fats and other stuff they add to them. Obviously, if you're always overdosing on carbohydrates, you will get fat, because the overwhelming excess energy will convert into body fat.

So what you should try to do is balance your intake of fuel with your need to burn it. Here's an 'idiot sheet' summarizing what you've learnt about carbohydrates:

- Carbohydrate foods have half the calories of fatty foods.
- You need carbohydrates for energy.
- You burn off carbohydrates when you exercise.
- Carbohydrates are a friendly fuel. Fat is your enemy.

Remember, when you're trying to lose weight, you need to eat the right quantities of high-grade carbohydrates. But make sure you eat less of the butter, mayonnaise, margarine and fatty sauces we associate with them.

Fats and carbohydrates

As we have seen, low GI carbohydrates are useful for controlling weight, but they can be negated by adding too much fat.

If you overuse fat it will end up being stored in your body in some way. You can actually calculate the fat content of packaged carbohydrates fairly simply. All carbohydrates have 4 calories per gram and fats have 9 calories per gram.

You can use the following calculation to see how the fat content of a product compares to its carbohydrate content. (It's a good idea to do this calculation when you buy something the first time and then you know what you're buying.) First, look at the product label. Then:

1. Multiply the total carbohydrate content (listed on the label) by 4 (i.e. calories per gram of carbohydrate).
2. Multiply the total fat content by 9 (i.e. calories per grams of fat).
3. Compare the two results as proportions of overall calories (or energy) of the product.

An example will help to clarify the process. Let's take a loaf of bread:

Example: bread

The label lists the following:

Typical values

	per 100 g	per slice
energy	300 kcal	100 kcal
protein	17.5 g	3.6 g
carbohydrates	50.0 g	20.3 g
(of which sugars)	5.0 g	2.1 g
fat	4.0 g	0.7 g
(of which saturates)	0.4 g	0.2 g
fibre	3.0 g	1.3 g
sodium	0.4 g	0.2 g

1. Multiply the total carbohydrate content of the product (50 grams) by 4 (calories per grams of carbohydrate):

$$50 \times 4 = 200 \text{ calories.}$$

2. Multiply the total fat content of the product (4 grams) by 9 (calories per grams of fat).

$$4 \times 9 = 36 \text{ calories.}$$

3. In 100 grams of this bread, there are 300 kcals of energy, of which 200 calories come from carbohydrates and 36 calories come from fats. So this bread has a low fat content.

If you remember, we said that 60 per cent of your food intake should be in the form of carbohydrates and 25 per cent should come from fats. In this case 66 per cent of the calories come from carbohydrates. (For the more technical among you, this figure is arrived at by dividing the carbohydrate calorific value of 200 by the total number of calories

> in 100 grams of the product and then multiplying by 100.)
> Twelve per cent came from fat. (Divide 36 by 300 and multi-
> ply by 100.)
>
> So the conclusion has to be that this product is a low-fat,
> high-carbohydrate item.

There are some hidden fats in carbohydrates, however, and you
won't necessarily know about them if the food has been prepared
in a restaurant or at a mate's house. But you should at least be
aware of them.

Of course, one individual item doesn't constitute a whole
meal's intake. This means you can eat a carbohydrate that has
slightly more fat than you would ideally like and balance it out
by adding salad, fruit and vegetables, which have a negligible fat
content.

The message here is that you should be aware of the calorific
values and fat content of food generally, but these must not
become a fixation like they do when you diet. When you meet a
strange piece of food for the first time, you can calculate its carbohydrate–fat ratio and then forget about it, because you know what
its value is. And there are benefits in knowing this stuff.

Energy conversion

If you still think that eating carbohydrates will make you gain
weight, consider this. Your body has to use up calories to convert
the carbohydrates you eat into energy. The cost of that process is
23 per cent of the available calories, so nearly a fifth of the kilo-
joules of the carbohydrates are used in digesting it. As a result,
your body converts carbohydrates into fat only in really unusual
circumstances, such as when you seriously overeat for ages at a
time.

Your body actually prefers the easy option and is far more eager
to add to your fat stores with the fats that you eat. Conversion of
the fat in food to energy is an extremely efficient process and uses
only 3 or 4 per cent of its value to digest it. Your body can thus go
on doing it virtually without limits. No matter how much fat you
eat, your body will go on faithfully storing it and turning it into
blubber.

Appetite satisfaction

In the old days people thought that proteins, fats and carbo-hydrates in equal quantities would satisfy the appetite equally. But recent research has found that the satiatory capacity of these three nutrients is not equal.

Fatty foods, in particular, are weak in satisfying hunger, so you tend to eat more high-fat foods just to stop being hungry. But high-carbohydrate, low-fat foods can be eaten till the appetite is satisfied. Because fat has over twice the calories of carbohydrates, apart from your body's natural desire to store fats as fat, you will tend to put on weight. Tests carried out in Australia found that high-quality carbohydrates, including potatoes, porridge, apples, pears and pasta, fill you much quicker than other major food groups. Eating more of these satisfies your appetite without adding calories.

On the other hand, high-fat foods that provide a lot of calories per gram, like croissants, chocolates and peanuts, were found to be the least satisfying. These make us store fat quicker and are less filling to eat. Unfortunately, although these kinds of foods disguise it and are delicious in the short term, they are bad for you.

Carbohydrates – top tips

- Use low GI carbohydrates as the mainstay of your daily intake. Two meals a day is about right, but you can use higher GI carbohydrates after a long period of exercise.
- Pay attention to the nutrient data on the side of food packets to see that the proportion of fat is not too high.
- Minimize the addition of fats to your carbohydrates.
- Eat enough carbohydrates to account for around 60 per cent of your food intake by calories. You can achieve this by eating the right number of servings, which you will find in the food pyramid.
- Carbohydrates are more filling that fatty foods and have fewer calories, so eat low-fat carbohydrates.
- Eat the right number and size of servings of grains, cereals, pasta, rice, vegetables and fruit, and you will take in the right amount of carbohydrate. Don't be tempted to cheat on portion sizes, because – unless you take much more exercise – you will put on weight.

7
Proteins

Before we ask how much protein we need and where we should get it from, it is important to understand the role protein plays in the structure and mechanisms of the body, and to find out what types of protein are available.

What does protein do?

Protein has two jobs. The first is structural. Structural proteins are found in the material of muscle, bone, hair, nails, skin, blood, connective tissue and other areas. The percentage content of these body parts varies, but whether it is large or small proportionately it is always essential.

The second job of protein is functional. Functional proteins are required in the formation and function of a variety of hormones, digestive enzymes and antibodies. Proteins are also found in the nuclei of cells (nucleoproteins) which transmit hereditary characteristics and so are responsible for continued protein synthesis within the cell.

In other words, proteins, and the amino-acids that make up proteins, are at the very core of our existence.

Where does protein come from?

Proteins are composed of long chains of building blocks called amino-acids. The sequence of these amino-acids determines the job a particular protein does, and its character. There are 20 or so amino-acids. About twelve of them can be synthesized by the body and are classed as non-essential types. The remaining eight have to come from the food we eat and these are classed as essential types.

Food which provides protein can be classified in two ways. The first is high-quality protein, a food type which supplies significant quantities of all eight essential amino-acids. Foods that do this are generally of animal origin, such as meat, fish and dairy products.

The second type is low-quality protein, supplying a proportion of the eight essential amino-acids. These foods are generally of vegetable origin.

It is possible, though, to combine two vegetable foods so that they form the eight essential amino-acids, making 'complete' protein. Vegetable protein or 'incomplete protein' can also be made into the complete type by combining it with an animal protein.

There are two ways of making complete protein. It was thought previously that either vegetable matter combinations or vegetable matter and animal protein combinations had to be consumed at the same meal. This is not true. Incomplete protein eaten at lunchtime can be mixed with complementary incomplete protein at dinner to make complete protein.

Unless you have enough complete protein you can't utilize it.

How much protein do I need?

By eating your pyramid serving groups you will get enough protein, the main sources being:

- two to four servings from the meat, poultry, fish, beans and nuts group
- two or three servings from the dairy group.

Any shortfall will be made up from incomplete proteins from the other groups. To check in a quantitative way, you can use the following method. The table below shows how much protein you as an individual should be eating per day, based on your own ideal set-point body weight (which you can calculate using the equation on page 33). These recommendations include a margin of safety and are approximations.

Fitness level of individual	Grams of protein per lb of body weight
adult recreational exerciser	0.5–0.75
adult exercising more than 5 hours per week	0.6–0.9
adult building muscle mass	0.7–0.9
maximum usable amount for adults	0.9

(Adapted from Nancy Clark, *Sports Nutrition Guidebook* [Human Kinetics, 1997])

Multiplying your weight in pounds by the key that fits your profile should give you an idea of your ideal daily protein intake.

In order to use this figure, you need to have a rough idea of the protein content per gram of different foods. Remember, 100 grams of meat don't contain 100 grams of protein, which is something people find confusing.

Use the following guidelines to calculate quantities of protein in grams.

- Each pyramid serving of meat, fish, poultry or beans gives you an average of 20 grams of protein.
- Each pyramid serving of dairy products gives you an average of 7 grams of protein (except cottage cheese, which is much higher at approximately 25 grams).

By adding the number of grams together you will get an approximation of your daily protein intake. Other food groups can be counted on to supply at least 20 per cent of your protein requirement, so you should allow for this as well. Don't worry yourself unduly about these figures, because the pyramid will take care of you. However, if you find it interesting, you might like to do it on occasion, especially if you are training hard and want to double-check you are getting enough protein.

Vegetarianism and protein

Vegetarianism can complicate the issue of getting enough usable complete protein. Protein is present in the main pyramid food groupings in varying quantities, but not all contain the eight essential amino-acids. The dairy and meat and fish sections do. The cereals, pasta, rice and vegetable and fruit sections do not. Vegetarians who do not eat dairy products, let alone meat or fish products, must therefore eat complementary vegetables, fruits and cereals, etc. to form complete protein.

There is some danger in this, because protein proportions are lower in these sections, so you do have to eat larger portions to get enough. You might get the protein requirement right, but eat more than the recommended number of serving portions and then find that your calorie intake is too high.

Vegetarians must be careful to consume vegetable/fruit/cereal/pasta/rice/grain/legume (pulse) combinations that have low-fat and high-protein quality. Some good options are listed below.

Grains and milk products (for lacto-vegetarians)

- cereal (low GI type) and milk (skimmed) or yoghurt
- pasta and low-fat cheese
- bread (low GI type) and low-fat cheese
- grains and beans and legumes (such as peanuts, chick-peas, lentils and beans)
- rice (non-sticky type) and beans
- pitta bread and split-pea soup
- bread and baked beans.

Legumes and seeds

Lacto-vegetarians are advised to eat:

- chick-peas and tahini (sesame paste)
- tofu and sesame seeds.

Vegetarians who go for dairy protein instead of meat or fish protein can have difficulties because dairy products can be high in fat. So care should be taken to use low-fat dairy products. By reading the nutrition labels on a product you can see whether it is low or high in fat.

To work out the fat percentage of a labelled product, you can use the following calculation:

1. Multiply the grams of fat by 9 (the number of calories in a gram of fat).
2. Divide this total by the number of calories per 100 grams to find out the percentage of fat.

Example: a 100 g pot of yoghurt

The yoghurt contains 85 calories and 4 grams of fat.

1. Multiply the grams of fat by 9 (the number of calories in a gram of fat) = 36 cals

2. To get the percentage, divide 36 by the number of calories in 100 g:
$$36 \div 85 = 0.42 \times 100 = 42 \%$$

So the fat content of this yoghurt (4 grams, or 42 per cent) is high. Some yoghurts have only 1 gram of fat.

Animal protein and fat

The reason it is worth talking specifically about protein from animal sources (dairy products and meat) is that some sources contain more fat than others. They also contain high proportions of saturated fat, which, eaten in excess, is bad for your health. So it is wise to know about these sources of protein. Animal protein should be looked at specifically in terms of its fat content. Here are some fat-content figures for animal protein:

Dairy products

	Grams of fat
milk (1 cup)	
regular	10
semi-skimmed	4
skimmed	0
yoghurt (200-g/7-oz tub)	
regular	10
fat free	0
ice cream (2 scoops)	
regular	10
skimmed	3
cheese	
Cheddar (30 g/1 oz)	10
reduced-fat Cheddar (30 g/1 oz)	3
low-fat processed (30 g/1 oz)	2.5
cottage cheese (2 tbsp)	4
ricotta (2 tbsp)	4
cream/sour cream (1 tbsp)	8

Meat

beef	
beef steak, lean only (75 g/3 oz)	10
minced beef (75 g/3 oz)	17
lean minced beef (75 g/3 oz)	16
beef frankfurter (75 g/3 oz)	25
lean rump steak, roasted (75 g/3 oz)	5.5
corned beef, canned (75 g/3 oz)	12.5
lamb	
lean chump chop, grilled (75 g/3 oz)	9
lean leg, roasted (2 slices)	5
2 lean loin chops	5

	Grams of fat
pork	
bacon, grilled (1 rasher)	9
lean ham (1 slice)	2
lean leg, roasted meat (3 slices)	4
loin chop, without fat	4
chicken	
chicken breast without skin, grilled (75 g/3 oz)	3
chicken breast with skin, grilled (75 g/3 oz)	7
chicken breast, poached and drained (75 g/3 oz)	2.5
chicken wing, roasted (75 g/3 oz)	9.5
fish	
cod, poached (75 g/3 oz)	0.75
herring, kippered (75 g/3 oz)	10.5
salmon, steamed (75 g/3 oz)	6.5
sardines, grilled (75 g/3 oz)	9.5
canned tuna in oil (75 g/3 oz)	7
canned tuna in brine (75 g/3 oz)	0.5
fish fingers, grilled (4)	12

Good animal protein low-fat choices

Based on the above figures, here are some suggestions to follow when eating animal protein products. By using these as the main-stay of your intake you will significantly lower your fat consumption. We recommend that you eat:

- chicken
- turkey
- fish
- skimmed milk
- low-fat cottage cheese (use this instead of butter)
- low-fat fromage frais
- low-fat yoghurt.

Protein – top tips

- Ensure that you get an adequate amount of complete protein from the animal, fish, poultry, dairy and beans sources. Top up from the vegetable grains and fruit groups.
- If you are a vegetarian, combine your incomplete protein sources to form complete protein. Try to use low GI carbohydrate types.
- Animal protein sources are high in saturated fats. Whenever possible, go for the lowest fat content available.
- Don't overdose on protein. Enough is enough. Any more will be stored as fat.

8
Fats

All through the protein and carbohydrates sections we've been talking about fats as one entity. Our simple message to you is that if you eat too much fat you will have a tendency to store it on your body and this will make you fat. Fat has twice as many calories as other food types, so it's a potent fuel.

But now it's time to go further and deeper into the subject. Fats can be broken down into saturated and unsaturated types and all foods with fats contain a mixture of these. It's the proportions that change.

I know what you're thinking: where's my list? Well, fear not, here is one.

Fats

	Saturates	Unsaturated
vegetable fats		
coconut oil	90 %	10 %
palm oil	50 %	50 %
animal fats		
butterfat	65 %	35 %
beef fat	50 %	50 %
chicken fat	30 %	70 %
Oils		
olive oil	15 %	85 %
canola oil	5 %	95 %
peanut oil	20 %	80 %
safflower oil	10 %	90 %
sunflower oil	10 %	90 %
corn oil	15 %	85 %

(Adapted from Nancy Clark, *Sports Nutrition Guidebook* [Human Kinetics, 1997])

The unsaturated fats are the good guys here and it is much more desirable to have them in your oils than saturated fats. If you want to really get on the case, you can break them down further into monounsaturated and polyunsaturated.

You can more or less categorize the saturated type of fats as being higher in animal-origin food and the two unsaturated types as higher in plant-origin food.

The fats that you find starring in a heart attack near you are the saturated kind. For the collector of gruesome facts, these include links with coronary heart disease, hypertension and arteriosclerosis.

Saturated animal fats are solid at room temperature. As your arteries operate at room temperature, it is easy to understand how this could translate into blockages in your system.

Some polyunsaturated fats (in the form of oil) are made into solid types by putting hydrogen through them. In this way they can be used in margarine. However, in some respects they then take on the form of saturated fats in terms of health. The use of partially hydrogenated fat produce should be minimized. Labelling on products will alert you to its presence. Choose margarine that has liquid oil as the first ingredient on its label.

Healthy proportions

When you eat fat, you take in both saturated and unsaturated types, but the proportions change. So you can veer towards the good types. A lot of labelling gives you both the gram quantity of total fats and the gram quantity of the saturated fats within that figure. Pay attention to product labels. If you get your fat intake approximately 25 per cent of your total calorie intake, this should be made up of equal proportions of saturated, monounsaturated and polyunsaturated fats. But that's hard to achieve in practice. Instead, aim to minimize your saturated fat intake and make the remainder up from the unsaturated types. This is realistic for day-to-day living.

Cholesterol

Cholesterol is a waxy substance that plays an essential part in the following:

- the functioning of your adrenal system (hormone production)
- metabolism of carbohydrates
- the manufacture of vitamin D from sunlight
- the composition of nerve fibre-sheaths.

Cholesterol can be manufactured by your body or ingested with your food. It is also a by-product of consuming saturated fat. As with a lot of substances in the body, enough is great, too much is a problem. Cholesterol is carried to where it is needed by lipoproteins. There are two types:

- low-density lipoproteins (LDL), which carry 60 per cent of blood cholesterol
- high-density lipoproteins (HDL), which carry 20 per cent of blood cholesterol.

If LDL types build up to dangerous levels once the body has used what it needs, the surplus has a tendency to stick to the artery walls. In time, this can become dangerous, contributing to heart disease through arterial blockage. Fortunately, HDL can help in that it will carry away the LDL type from these areas like a vacuum cleaner and take it back to the liver for disposal.

Unsaturated and omega 3 fats (a type of polyunsaturated fat found in some fish) help in the removal of LDL deposits. This is why they are recommended over saturated types of fats, which are themselves linked with heightened cholesterol levels.

The omega 3 fats found in some cold-water fish should be eaten a couple of times a week to reduce the effect of the LDL cholesterol. Fish such as salmon, mackerel, tuna, sardines and herring are recommended. Supplements are also available, but they are not as potent. A 100-gram (4-oz) piece of tuna equals ten pills of a normal fish-oil supplement. Vegetarians might need to take these supplements, but their cholesterol level is probably not an issue because of their reduced saturated-fat intake.

Another way to reduce cholesterol is to eat foods low in the substance, or at least stay away from those that are high in it.

At present it is not certain that some foods automatically raise cholesterol to harmful levels. Eggs, though high in the substance, seem to affect different people differently. The American Heart Association recommends an intake of 300 mg a day, and to be safe, especially if you have a genetic disposition to high cholesterol levels, this seems a good idea. (By the way, a food labelled 'low cholesterol' means it is not more than 20 mg a serving.)

To reduce high cholesterol (LDL) levels, do regular aerobic exercise. An hour and a half a week will reduce it by 10 per cent.

Cholesterol content

	Amount	Cholesterol (mg)
milk		
skimmed	1 cup	5
semi-skimmed	1 cup	10
whole	1 cup	35
eggs	1	210
cheese		
Cheddar	1oz	30
mozzarella	1oz	15
ricotta	half a cup	40
cottage cheese (low-fat)	half a cup	5
ice cream, full-fat	100 g	44
ice cream, low-fat	100 g	10–20
lean meat and fish (cooked)		
beef liver	100 g (3½ oz)	482
Kentucky fried chicken	100 g (3½ oz)	76
chicken breast	100 g (3½ oz)	95
lamb	100 g (3½ oz)	100
pork	100 g (3½ oz)	85
tuna, canned	100 g (3½ oz)	45
shrimps	100 g (3½ oz)	175 g

(Adapted from Nancy Clark, *Sports Nutrition Guidebook* [Human Kinetics, 1997])

This will make your HDL (good cholesterol) levels go up and make you lose weight, which inhibits the effect of LDL types.

Soluble fibre, the type found in beans, legumes, oat bran and pectin, also lowers bad cholesterol and should be included as part of a healthy eating plan. Tests have shown that moderate amounts of this fibre can decrease your risk of heart disease by significant percentages. Other cholesterol-reducing foods are garlic and evening primrose oil. A glass of red wine a day is also good for this. (Hurrah!)

Low fat, what does it mean?

Some foods are naturally low in fat. Others are naturally high in fat, but their fat content has been reduced. Sometimes this is confusing, so read the product label to help you work it out.

Remember, whether a product is described as half-fat, reduced-fat or low-fat, it still contains fat, and the appropriate question to ask is not whether it has less fat, but what the original fat content was. A product can be reduced in fat but still be a high-fat food. So you need to be able to read food nutrition labels.

Say you are attempting to obtain 25 per cent of your calories from fats. Look at the calorie/gram quantity of fat on the label as a percentage of the total energy/calorie quantity of 100 grams of the product. This will give you some idea of the actual fat content. Use the following method as a basis for your calculations.

For example, say 100 grams of fish contains 200 calories. Within those 100 grams, there are 4 grams of fat.

1. Multiply the fat content by 9 (the number of calories in a gram of fat):

$$4 \times 9 \text{ calories} = 36 \text{ calories}$$

2. Divide this result by the total calories/energy of the product:

$$36 \div 200 = 0.18$$

3. Multiply this result by 100:

$$0.18 \times 100 = 18 \text{ \%}$$

The final result – 18 per cent – is well within your 25 per cent limit.

If you then fry the fish, the percentage will go up because of the added fat for cooking. If you grill it or poach it, the fat content will actually be reduced.

These methods of calculating fat are OK if not overdone. I find them of interest, but no more than that. A better way is to cut down on fatty foods as a general rule, but within moderation. Remember, you need a minimum of 30 to 40 grams (about 1½ ounces) of fat a day even if you are in weight-loss mode.

Fats added to natural foods will obviously increase your fat intake. If you are not careful, you can end up with more grams of fat than you need.

Fat content

	Calories
butter/margarine (1 tsp)	36
oil, any type (1 tbsp)	120
cooking spray (per spray)	9
mayonnaise (1 tbsp)	63
salad dressing (1 tbsp)	45

Cooking oil in spray form is a good idea because it is controllable.

How much fat should I eat in a day?

less than 40 grams	*Excellent* 30–40 grams (1½ oz) is amount of fat you should be eating per day if you're aiming to lose body fat.
41–60 grams	*Good* A fat intake in this range is recommended for most adult men and women who are maintaining their body weight
61–80 grams	*Acceptable* If you are working out very hard or your work is very labour intensive. It is too much if you are trying to lose weight.
More than 80 grams	*Unacceptable* You are probably eating too much fat.

If you are in the lower limits of the serving numbers within the food pyramid, you will be eating about 1400–1600 calories a day. If your daily fat intake is 40 grams (about 1½ ounces), 360 calories come from fat. Divide this figure by 1500, then multiply by 100 to get the percentage:

$$360 \div 1500 = 0.24 \%$$

The result – 24 per cent – is about right.

Cooking tips to reduce fat intake

- Grill, poach or steam as opposed to frying or roasting foods.

- Spray, rather than pour, oils.

- Potatoes and vegetable purées can be used to thicken sauces, stews and pie contents rather than flour and butter. They are also higher in vitamins and minerals. Purée the vegetables and then add stock as required.

- If you're preparing gravy, do it early and then refrigerate it. You can then skim off in one lump the saturated fat (the main fat in meats) that will form on top.

- Use herbs to season dishes that are low in fat. This will help overcome the loss of flavour that comes from reducing fat content.

- Experiment with whole grains like millet, kasha and barley to give body to meals without high fat content.

- Cook rice with a little fruit juice and lots of herbs. You can even add alcohol, as most of the sugar it contains will disappear during cooking. *Don't* add any oil.

- When cooked, enrich mashed potatoes with an egg. Eggs have less fat than the butter and cream normally added to mashed potatoes.

- Use balsamic vinegar, mustard and a tablespoon of soft tofu to make a low-fat dressing for salads. Lose the oil, or minimize it.

- Get a good non-stick frying-pan and you will not need so much oil. You can fry an egg without any extra fat if you have a good frying-pan.

- Grilling vegetables with a little oil spray is much better than frying them. It also enhances their flavour.

- Fat-free or low-fat marinades are a good way of flavouring foods without using oils. You can cook the food with the marinades as well.

- Cream toppings tend to be used to tone down the sweetness of desserts. Make a less sweet dessert and eliminate the need for cream, or use low-fat yoghurt or fromage frais instead.

- Transform vinaigrette into a smooth and creamy dressing by adding low- or non-fat yoghurt or cottage cheese.

- Curry powder and/or chilli powder are so strong-tasting that they can hide the fact that the fat content of a food has been reduced.

- Remove fats from fish or animal meat foods, i.e. white fat from meats, the skin from chicken, turkey, duck and goose, and the white lumps from raw salmon (choose salmon that has as little white fat as possible).

- If you do roast foods (unavoidable sometimes), make sure that they're on a raised rack so the fat drops away as opposed to being reabsorbed.

- The cholesterol and fat in an egg is in the yolk. Most recipes are not dramatically changed if you halve the yolk content. You can make scrambled eggs with three egg whites and one yolk. With lots of herbs it tastes pretty good.

- De-fat your cheese. If you are using Cheddar or mozzarella cheese in a recipe, stick it in the microwave on full for two minutes. Then drain off the fat that forms on top. You get the cheese flavour but cut the fat content dramatically.

- As a general rule, if you are reducing your overall fat intake, ensure you maximize on other flavours or you will get bored and return to bad habits.

Fat – top tips

- Minimize your saturated fat intake and keep your total fat intake down to reasonable levels (about 35 grams/1½ ounces) a day in weight-loss mode and 40–60 grams/about 2 ounces at other times.

- Do not become obsessive about monitoring fat intake. You need it – it's just that you don't need too much of it.

- If you normally cook with a lot of oil, look at the fat-reducing cooking tips seriously. They will help.

9

Vitamins, Minerals and Liquids

Vitamins

Vitamins are metabolic catalysts which regulate bio-mechanical reactions within your body. So far thirteen have been discovered. Each has a specific function. The recommended daily allowances (RDA) for vitamins are set above the minimum required level in order to overcome conditions that may occur in a shortfall and provide a safety factor. For example, the amount of vitamin C that prevents the deficiency disease scurvy is 10 milligrams a day, but the RDA is 60 milligrams, six times the minimum amount. Using the pyramid food plan will provide the correct quantities of your daily vitamin needs. The vitamin content of food depends on its quality and freshness, and is affected by cooking methods.

Fat-soluble vitamins

Some vitamins are ingested via the fat we eat. These are not needed every day because they're stored in the liver and fat cells or body fat. Eating a diet with a fat intake lower than 20 grams (3/4 ounce) a day can lead to deficiencies of these vitamins. Fat intake is a very important part of a healthy eating regime. The fat-soluble vitamins are vitamins A, D, E and K. Each has a specific function and RDA. The table below will show you what you need and where to get it.

Vitamin breakdown

Vitamin	Recommended intake (RDA)	Functions	Sources
A (retinol)	5000 IU	necessary for healthy eyes and skin and linings of the digestive tracts and the nose	vitamin A can be manufactured in the body from beta carotene, which is widely found in green vegetables; retinol is present in milk, butter, cheeses and fortified margarines

Vitamin	Recommended intake (RDA)	Functions	Sources
B$_1$ (thiamin)	1.5 mg	helps transform carbohydrates into energy	cereals, enriched rice, bread, pork, eggs, bananas, legumes, fish and chicken
B$_2$ (riboflavin)	1.7mg	necessary for energy release and healthy skin, mucous membranes and nervous system	steak, dairy products, green leafy vegetables, enriched breads and cereals
B$_3$ (niacin)	20 mg	helps transform food into energy; necessary for growth and for production of hormones	liver, lean meats, fish, bread, cereals, corn, peas, tuna, whole grains and legumes
B$_6$ (pyridoxamine)	2.0 mg	necessary for synthesis of breakdown of amino-acids; aids in metabolism	meats, vegetables, whole-grain cereals and beans
folic acid (folate)	0.4 mg	necessary for production of blood cells and healthy nervous system	legumes, green vegetables and whole-wheat products
biotin	0.3 mg	needed for metabolism of carbohydrates, fats and proteins	legumes, vegetables and meats
pantothenic acid	10 mg	needed for metabolism of carbohydrates, fats and proteins	nuts, fish, meats, eggs, vegetables and whole wheat
B$_{12}$	6.0 mcg	needed for synthesis of red and white blood cells and metabolism of food	muscle meats, eggs and dairy products
C (ascorbic acid)	60 mg	necessary for healthy connective tissue, bones, teeth and cartilage; enhances immune system	citrus fruits, tomatoes, green peppers and salad greens
D (cholecalciferol)	400 iu	needed for calcium and phosphorous metabolism and for healthy bones and teeth	the sun's rays, cod liver oil, dairy products, fortified milk and margarine
E (tocopherol)	30 iu	necessary for nourishing and strengthening cells	seeds, green leafy vegetables; small amount in cereals, fruits and meats
K	70–140 mcg	necessary for blood clotting	green leafy vegetables; some in cereals, fruits and meats

Key

iu = international unit   mg = milligram   mcg = microgram

Water-soluble vitamins

Some vitamins are transported via the watery mediums in our bodies, and are stored in tissue. These must be consumed regularly, usually daily or at least within a period of several days. Water-soluble vitamins include vitamin C (ascorbic acid) and the B-complex groups: thiamin (B_1), riboflavin (B_2), niacin, pyroxidine (B_6), cobalamin (B_{12}), panothenic acid, folic acid and biotin. Their RDA sources can be found in the vitamin list.

Antioxidants

The current buzzword in vitamins is antioxidants. These are the vitamins A, C and E and they are found in fruits, vegetables and other wholesome foods. They can reduce the risk of heart disease by inhibiting oxidation of the bad type of cholesterol (LDL). Studies of both men and women have shown that those who took about 100 iu of vitamin E daily for at least 2 years had a 40 per cent lower risk of heart disease.

Antioxidants may also reduce the risk of developing cancer tumours. They appear to inhibit the natural process known as oxidation that can lead to the formation of potentially cancerous cells.

By eating a healthy diet, high in fruit and vegetables, you should be getting enough antioxidants. However, if you're worried that factors in your life conspire to reduce this intake, get a good multivitamin containing the antioxidant vitamins to make sure.

Can I get all my vitamin needs from food?

The short answer is yes. Having a healthy eating regime is the basis for ensuring correct vitamin intake, although factors such as modern food manufacturing, rushed or missed meals and a stressful lifestyle can upset your vitamin intake. Supplements are a valid solution, but you should always try to get the majority of your needs from food. In situations like those listed below you may need supplements:

- Restricted calorific intake
  The less calories you eat the more difficult it is to ensure your vitamin intake is sound. When in weight-loss mode, a high-quality multivitamin is a good idea.

- **Allergies to certain foods**
  People who cannot eat certain types of foods, such as fruit or wheat, need to compensate with alternative vitamin sources to avoid deficiencies in some nutrients.

  Lactose intolerance, or the inability to digest milk or dairy product sugar, can lead to deficiencies in riboflavin and calcium. Other foods can supply these vitamins and minerals, but to be safe a supplement is advisable.

- **Pregnancy**
  Expectant mothers require additional vitamins, and their doctors often recommend supplements. Women contemplating pregnancy are often advised to eat a diet rich in folic acid, or to take a multivitamin with 400 micrograms of folic acid. This B vitamin helps to prevent damage to the foetus at the time of conception and in the first twelve weeks of pregnancy.

- **Total vegetarians**
  People who abstain from eating any animal foods may become deficient in vitamins B_{12}, D and riboflavin. Those who eat a poorly balanced vegetarian diet can become deficient in protein, iron and zinc.

- **Illness**
  Illness can rob us of vitamins, a situation exacerbated by the medicinal drugs used in treatment.

- **Smoking and heavy drinking**
  These habits can contribute to specific vitamin deficiencies, particularly vitamin C. Supplements can be beneficial. Every cigarette you smoke destroys 25 milligrams of vitamin C.

- **Food manufacture and processing**
  Manufacturers want to provide food that is tasty, easy to prepare, looks good on the supermarket shelf and can be stored for a long time. But this can rob the food of vitamins. Apart from white flour and margarine, no foods are covered by laws to make manufacturers replace the nutrients destroyed during processing and refining. So be aware that highly processed foods can be low in vitamin content and that by eating from these sources you could end up with deficiencies.

How to choose a supplement

The market is flooded with vitamin and mineral supplements. To avoid confusion, if you feel you need a supplement, here are some ideas to help you choose:

- Choose a good multivitamin, the best you can afford.
- Don't go for the megadose variety. Anything above 1000 per cent RDA of a vitamin or mineral is too large and should not be regarded as a standard. (Doses are given on the packaging.)
- Choose vitamins with around 100 per cent of the RDA.
- Choose a multivitamin with beta-carotene, not vitamin A. Beta-carotene is used to make vitamin A, but also acts as an antioxidant.
- Natural or synthesized vitamins are the same, except for vitamin E (and even then the potency difference is minimal).
- Buy a multivitamin that has passed the 45-minute dissolution test. A supplement is of little use unless your body can absorb it.

Take your multivitamins with or after a meal. Store them in a cool, dry place and don't keep them beyond their expiry date.

How can we maximize natural vitamins from our food?

Eating the right food doesn't necessarily mean you are getting enough vitamins. They are easily killed by food processing, storing and cooking. To get the most from what you eat, keep the following in mind:

- Wash but don't soak fresh vegetables; otherwise vitamins B and C are destroyed.
- Prepare fruit and vegetables just before you eat them. If you leave them standing for more than a short period, a large percentage of the vitamins is lost.
- Over-storage causes vitamin loss. Green vegetables lose 10 per cent of their vitamin C content daily. An opened carton or bottle of orange juice will lose its vitamin C potency in a few days, less accelerated by shaking.
- Cooking in copper pots can destroy vitamin C, folic acid and vitamin E.
- The shortest cooking time and the smallest amount of water are the least destructive to vitamins.
- Use cooking water from vegetables and juices from meats to make soups.

- Light destroys vitamin A and B$_2$ over a period. Make sure your beta-carotene containing vegetables are kept dark and that milk bottles are removed from light sources after delivery.
- Keeping food warm for long periods induces general vitamin loss: 75 per cent can be lost if a meal is kept waiting for a few hours. The quicker a meal moves from kitchen to table the better.
- Store vegetables and fruit in the refrigerator as soon as you bring them home.
- Aluminium, stainless steel, glass and enamel are the best utensils for retaining nutrients while cooking. Iron pots can give you the benefit of that mineral, but they will short-change you on Vitamin C.
- To preserve the maximum amount of vitamins available from fruit and vegetables, eat them raw. (This ties in well with our plan to eat two to three snacks a day between meals because these can be when you eat your raw fruit and vegetables.)
- Do not use baking soda when cooking vegetables if you want to benefit from their thiamine and vitamin C.
- Most vitamins in fruit and vegetables are found in the outer layers, so try and peel sparingly or scrub instead where possible.
- Don't chop up vegetables and fruits too early before using as vitamin loss is substantial whilst they lie around.
- When you cut vegetables with a knife a substance is released from the ruptured cells which destroys vitamin C. Boiling excessively chopped vegetables increases the surface area in contact with the water, so losses are increased.

Minerals

Minerals, like vitamins, are essential for health. Some vitamins can be synthesized, but minerals are obtained solely from food. Minerals are more stable than vitamins and harder to destroy, but can still be lost during food refining, processing and cooking. In addition, minerals can be immobilized by other food factors and made unavailable to the body.

Minerals are grouped into two classes, according to the quantity needed by the body. Those required in doses higher than 100 milligrams a day are called macro-minerals; those required in smaller doses are known as trace minerals or elements. Some are needed in such tiny amounts, their requirements are measured in micrograms.

Minerals provide structure in the formation of bones and teeth. They have a functional role in maintaining normal heart rhythm, muscle contractility, nerve conduction and the body's acid base fluid balance. Minerals are essential for synthesis of the major biologic nutrients: glycogen from glucose, fats from fatty acids and glycerol and proteins from amino-acids. Minerals also form important constituents of hormones such as thyroxin and insulin.

They play a regulatory role in cellular metabolism and form an important part of enzymes and hormones that modify and regulate cellular hormones.

Where do I get the minerals I need?

The minerals required by the body can be readily obtained from food sources in a well-balanced diet. The mineral table below shows individual minerals and their most readily available source. Cutting out a major food type, like dairy products, will affect calcium mineral intake, so alternative sources from other foodstuffs should be found. You could also use a calcium supplement. If you still are unsure about your intake, consider taking a mineral supplement to make up any shortfall.

Macro-mineral and micro-mineral sources and RDA for adults aged 19–50

Macro-minerals

	RDA (mg)	Dietary sources	Major body functions
calcium	800	milk, cheese, dark green vegetables and dried legumes	bone and tooth formation, blood clotting and nerve transmission
phosphorous	800	milk, cheese, yoghurt, meat, poultry, grains and fish	bone and tooth formation; acid base balance
potassium	2000	leafy vegetables, cantaloupe melon, lima beans, potatoes, bananas, milk, meat, coffee and tea	fluid balance, nerve transmission and acid base balance
sulphur	unknown	obtained as part of dietary protein and is present in food preservatives	acid base balance and liver function

	RDA (mg)	Dietary sources	Major body functions
sodium	1100–3300	common salt	acid base balance, body water balance and nerve function
chlorine	700	chloride is part of self-containing food; occurs in some vegetables and fruit	important part of extra-cellular fluids
magnesium	350 (men) 280 (women)	whole grains and green leafy vegetables	activates enzymes involved in protein synthesis
Micro-minerals			
iron	10 (men) 15 (women)	eggs, lean meats, legumes, whole grains and green leafy vegetables	constituent of blood and enzymes involved in energy metabolism
fluorine	1.5–4.0 (average value)	drinking water, tea and seafood	may be important in maintenance of bone structure
zinc	15 (men) 12 (women)	widely distributed in foods	constituent of enzymes involved in digestion
copper	1.5–3.0 (average value)	meats and drinking water	constituent of enzymes
selenium	0.070 (men) 0.055 (women)	seafood, meat and grains	functions in close association with vitamin E
iodine	150	marine fish and shellfish, dairy products, vegetables and iodized salt	constituent of thyroid hormones
chromium	0.075–0.25 (men) 0.05–0.25 (women) (average values)	legumes, cereals, organ meats, fats, vegetable oils, meats and whole grains	constituent of some enzymes involved in glucose and energy metabolism

Iron and zinc

Iron and zinc are both more readily absorbed from animal sources than from vegetable sources. It you are a vegetarian, select breads and cereals with the words 'iron enriched' or 'iron fortified' on the label. This will increase the small amounts of iron available from the grain. Think about taking a multimineral supplement.

The list below shows the iron and zinc content of different foods.

	iron (mg)	zinc (mg)
Animal sources		
beef (110 g/4 oz)	3	6
turkey, dark meat (110 g/4 oz)	2	5
pork (110 g/4 oz)	1	3
oysters, raw (6 medium)	6	75
shrimp (12 large)	2	1
chicken breast (110 g/4 oz)	1	1
chicken liver, cooked (110 g/4 oz)	9	5
haddock (110 g/4 oz)	1	1
tuna, light (85 g/3 oz)	1	1
eggs (1 large)	1	0.5
Fruit and juice sources		
prune juice	3	0.5
apricots (5 halves)	0.8	0.3
dates, dried (10)	1	0.2
raisins (1 cup)	3	0.3
Vegetable and legume sources		
refried beans (1 cup)	4.5	3.5
spinach, cooked (half a cup)	3	1
tofu (1 cake)	8	4
peas (1 cup)	2	2
broccoli (1 cup)	2	0.6
Dairy sources		
skimmed milk (1 cup)	0.1	1.0
Cheddar cheese (25 g/1 oz)	0.2	1.0
Grain sources		
cereal (1 cup)	18	0.7
Raisin bran (1 cup)	24	5.3
cream of wheat (1 cup)	9	0.3

(Adapted from Nancy Clark, *Sports Nutrition Guidebook* [Human Kinetics, 1997])

Minerals – top tips

- Go for mineral nutrition through healthy, nutritious, mineral-rich food. If you're vegetarian, think about getting the minerals iron and zinc from supplements or eating foods with especially rich iron in them on a regular basis.
- If you don't eat any dairy products either eat other calcium-rich foods or take a calcium supplement.
- Use cast-iron cooking pots. A cast-iron pot used over a period of three months to cook spaghetti sauce increases the iron content of the food dramatically (from 3 to 88 milligrams).
- Avoid coffee and tea: they decrease iron absorption.

- Zinc absorption is increased when vitamin A, calcium and phosphorus are taken at the same time, but its absorption can be interfered with by a number of other nutrients. It has been suggested that taking a zinc supplement last thing at night on an empty stomach can raise absorption levels.
- Remember, mineral supplements are available, but don't take more than the RDA.
- Iron and zinc are absorbed best from animal sources (except for iron in eggs).

Liquids

In this section I want to talk mainly about water, but it's worth mentioning alcohol, coffee, tea and fizzy drinks.

Water

Most of your body is made up of water. We sweat in order to balance the heat generated from bodily processes. When we exercise we sweat a lot, because we get hot. When we urinate and defecate to get rid of bodily waste, we also get rid of a lot of water. Think of your body as a water tower with a slow leak; if you don't keep topping up you eventually run out.

Water is central to most of our bodily processes. Without correct levels of water you can't digest properly (because of insufficient saliva), exercise efficiently (because water transports glucose to muscles), keep your metabolism at an optimum level, or metabolize fat, for example. You can live for weeks without food, but only three or four days without water.

The food we eat contains different proportions of water. Juicy fruits are some of the high-content ones, meat and eggs to a lesser extent. Drinks such as coffee, tea and alcohol are all water-based. The easiest way to give your body enough water is to drink it plain. Mineral waters are generally better, but tap water is OK unless you live in urban areas, in which case you should filter it.

The quantity you drink a day depends on your exercise levels. As a rule of thumb six or seven glasses spread over a day and especially before, during and after exercise is about right, but increase this if you do a long run or some other form of strenuous, sweaty exercise.

Water is also a great filler and drinking it in the evening can stop you reaching for the biscuits. Richard is a great believer in soup as a snack, particularly late at night, basically because it's low

GI and also bangs hunger on the head. It's the water content and volume of the soup that does it.

The Parachute Regiment used to practise water conservation by being allowed only a couple of sips of water an hour while they were fast marching. The purpose was to teach them the importance of not wasting water. Although it was a useful lesson, it had a major flaw: soldiers kept going down with heat-stroke, some badly. You can easily die of it. Low water intake, even if to a lesser degree, can affect you adversely. So, drink water.

An easy way to check if you're dehydrated is to count how many times you urinate in a day (the optimum is about five to eight times), check how much you urinate each time (the more the better), and observe the colour of your urine. The darker the colour, the more likely you are dehydrated because the coloured waste products are more concentrated.

Coffee and tea

Coffee and tea with sugar can play havoc with your blood sugar levels. If you take sugar in your tea you are, over a day, taking five or six teaspoons of pure cane sugar. This can significantly raise your blood sugar levels, especially if you've just eaten, because your levels will have already gone up from the food calories. This will instigate the release of insulin, with the resultant drop in blood sugar, and an hour later you'll feel tired and listless because your levels will have plummeted.

If you drink more tea or coffee, the whole cycle begins again. So reduce or give up the sugar and drink less tea and coffee. Exactly the same principle applies to fizzy sugary drinks but even more so. There are more than four teaspoons of sugar in a can of Coke. The caffeine content of these products is addictive and energy-sapping, too.

I buy the best-quality decaffeinated tea or coffee I can afford and savour it as a treat twice a day rather than hourly. And I don't use sugar any more. Try it.

Alcohol

Alcohol contains seven calories per gram, two calories less than fat, but three more than protein or carbohydrate. It doesn't have any great nutritional value. Red wine can help reduce cholesterol, but then again so can lots of other things. The higher the percentage proof of alcohol in a product, the more calories it has, so spirits are very high calorifically.

All alcoholic drinks are high on the glycaemic index (beer is 110) so its energy releases large amounts of sugar very quickly into the bloodstream, causing insulin overdoses. And we know that's undesirable. It doesn't provide much usable energy in carbohydrate form either. That said, it is nice. But it's a matter of balance (especially after a few pints). In health terms, alcohol really doesn't have much to offer. Go for it if you enjoy it, but cut down. And never drink alcohol because you're thirsty. Drink water first to kill your thirst and then alcohol for fun.

We recommend that you stop drinking altogether when you want to maximize body-fat loss. Otherwise, a glass or two of wine two or three times a week is probably the best option, and it's certainly preferable to beer or spirits. If you drink too much at a party, mentally compute that a couple of aerobic sessions will redress the balance. But don't try to do it all in one go, because alcohol dehydrates you. It mixes very badly with hard exercise and can be dangerous.

Sports drinks

Sports drinks make great claims about enhancing sports performance. If you eat balanced nutritious meals and drink water throughout the day, especially before, during and after exercise, these other drinks do little more for you. If you drink them before exercise, the sugar content can actually reduce your stamina and performance. At the levels most people exercise (an hour to an hour and a half), you're better off drinking water and eating a potassium-rich banana to redress your blood sugar balance and to rehydrate. Its cheaper and better for you.

Liquids – top tips

- Drink lots of water, at least six or seven glasses a day – more if you are exercising aerobically for long periods.
- Drink high-quality coffee and tea (decaff preferably), but limit it to two or three cups of either a day.
- Alcohol – if you enjoy it too much to give up, try to limit your intake to a couple of glasses of white wine two or three times a week maximum. If you drink spirits, give serious thought to stopping.
- Sports drinks are OK, but for cheapness and a similar effect eat a banana and drink lots of water.

10
Food Rules

We lead busy lives and our eating habits can be sporadic. We are adversely affected by what we eat, when we eat and how much we eat. This has a greater effect on us than we think. If we adhere to the calorie theory of eating it shouldn't really matter whether we have one very large meal a day or five smaller meals as long as they balance in calorie content. In fact, the opposite is true, however. The reasons tie in with everything we've been saying throughout the book about blood sugar levels, insulin release, raising metabolic levels and the way the body regenerates itself in the muscle department. So it's a good idea to look at the structure of the way we eat to get the best out our food. These rules will help you structure how you eat and decide to do it our way. (Or we'll send the boys round to your place.)

Rules

1. Eat regularly throughout the day, including three main meals and at least two snacks.
2. Your main meals should get smaller as the day goes on, ending with a simple evening meal.
3. Be organized with the type of food you keep in the house and the food you order in restaurants.
4. Keep a food diary, even if it's only in your head.
5. Maintain some balance in your attitude to food management. Don't panic.

Rule 1

Eat regularly throughout the day, including three main meals and at least two snacks.

The purposes of this rule are:

- to maintain your blood sugar levels at an optimum level throughout the day,

- to keep your metabolism on the hop from the moment you awake till the moment you fall asleep.

Your blood sugar needs to be kept at the mid-point between being too low (hypoglycaemic) and too high (hyperglycaemic). Then your body works efficiently. Your thought processes are clear and alert, your mood is generally relaxed and you won't be getting any severe hunger signals. If you eat in a way that accomplishes this with small movements of your blood sugar up and down you will find that life becomes much easier and less frantic. Your blood sugar level is dictated by the foods you eat and the food you don't eat.

If you miss meals, you will get low blood sugar at some stage. If you then catch up on your missed meals by having a major 'chow down', the size or quantity of the meal will raise your blood sugar levels. This will lead to an eating pattern that buggers up your life. So eat little and often.

Starting with breakfast, you should eat something about every two and a half hours. Between main meals this can be a snack, which is a useful nutritional tool. Richard makes his clients eat at least 30 per cent of their daily intake raw (and they pay him for this – astonishing).

Snacks are great for covering the raw side of eating. Choose a piece of fruit (low GI, of course) or some vegetable you like. Or, on occasion, a low GI carbohydrate like a cup of lentil soup or a Ryvita with some low-fat cottage cheese. These snacks give you sustained energy till you reach your main meal. Eat high GI food as a snack and you won't get the sustained energy so choose carefully. Here's the sugar day from hell neatly laid out for you:

07.30   Get up.

08.00   Breakfast – missed it, too busy and late for work.

10.00   Mid-morning. Really hungry and rather tired. (This is because your blood sugar levels are getting lower and lower. Your last meal was last night, so no wonder.) Eventually go out and buy some chocolate and a cup of coffee. Feel better for an hour, then feel tired again. (This is because the sugar in the chocolate has made you release a large dose of insulin which trashes your blood sugar levels to an even lower level.)

11.30	Look forward to lunch, but keep drinking coffee to keep going.
13.00	Pub. Eat dodgy-looking sandwich with a couple of pints. (This sends your blood sugar up again – beer is very high GI – with the inevitable 'crash' in the afternoon, making you feel sleepy.)
14.00	Try to concentrate all afternoon but find it difficult. Still feeling hungry, so nibble biscuits.
17.00	Try to catch up with work. Decide to eat out on the way home. Have a curry and couple of lagers. (By this stage your blood sugar levels are going up and down like a yo-yo. Your brain keeps receiving conflicting signals of hunger when your blood sugar is low and anxiety and irritability when it's high. Your body is storing calories very readily because of the heightened presence of insulin in your system. In a word, you are 'unbalanced'.)
23.00	Go to bed feeling rather tired and unsettled. (The curry you ate contained loads of fat, so your body has to work overtime to deal with it. There's a mountain of energy flowing round your system with nothing to do and, with this sort of imbalance in your system, when you wake up you'll probably repeat the whole cycle again.)

So what's a better way? The next diary is for a day based on the following serving numbers, suitable for an average-sized man:

Food group	Servings
dairy	2 1/2
meat, fish, poultry, beans, nuts	2 1/2
vegetables	4
fruit	3
cereals, grains, pasta, rice	8

07.00	Get up. Drink a glass of water. Do stretching exercises.
07.30–08.00	Have breakfast consisting of: 225 g (8 oz) low-fat yoghurt – dairy, 1 serving 60 g (2 oz) All Bran cereal – cereals, grains, etc., 3 servings

100 ml (4 oz) skimmed milk – dairy, half a serving
$^1/_2$ medium grapefruit – fruit, 1 serving
1 cup of tea
1 cup of water

09.30–10.30   Get to work and work steadily till lunchtime.
Have a snack:
an apple – fruit, 1 serving
stick of celery – vegetables, 1 serving
1 cup of water

13.00   Go to Italian restaurant. Have the following meal:
85 g (3 oz) pasta – cereals, grains, etc., 3 servings
three-quarters of a cup tomato-based sauce –
    vegetable, 1 serving
1 cup mineral water
Work all afternoon; get a lot done.

16.00   Have snack to keep going:
half a piece of Ryvita – cereals, grains, etc., half a
    serving
1 cup cottage cheese – dairy, 1 serving
a peach – fruit, 1 serving

17.00   Stop for a cup of tea.

18.00–19.00   Go to the gym. Drink 2 glasses of water before,
during and after session.

19.30   Eat easy-to-prepare meal of:
170 g (6 oz) marinated chicken – meat, poultry, etc.,
    2 servings
half a cup of broccoli – vegetables, 1 serving
half a mixed salad – vegetables, 1 serving
1 small whole-grain roll – cereals, grains, etc.,
    1 serving
1 cup of water

20.00–22.00   Work for a couple of hours.

22.00   Go to bed.

Throughout this day you fed your body what it needed to keep going without overloading or starving it. The calorific value of the evening meal above is approximately 1600–1800 calories, which is fine for a medium-sized man who is trying to lose some body fat.

Your metabolism

Your metabolism is changeable and can be affected in a number of ways that won't serve your needs. When you miss meals, your metabolism has a tendency to slow down. You're sending it messages that food is scarce, so it will attempt to get more from the food you do give it. A pattern of eating where you don't eat much during the day and then eat a lot at night will do just that. Not good.

By eating a lot of food in one go you overload your digestive system, which not only makes you feel unwell, with an acid stomach, but also overworks your digestive system. This slows down your metabolism. The calorific energy it takes to digest five light meals is greater than that required for, say, two very large meals. This means you're expending more energy in digesting your food, but you're doing it in a way that your body copes with more easily. This is good metabolism-raising stuff.

Eating little and often can be complicated. Sometimes you have to miss lunch or a snack. If you do miss lunch, keep snacking every two and a half hours until you can get a main meal.

Rule 2

Your main meals should get smaller and simpler as the day goes on, ending with a simple evening meal.

The saying goes: 'Breakfast like a king, lunch like a prince and dine like a pauper.' It's good advice. The majority of energy is used during working hours and food intake should be geared towards fuelling it. A major mistake we make nowadays is that we do the reverse. We eat very little during the day and then eat loads in the evening. So the energy we are making has nowhere to go.

Your body regenerates at night, it does it just as well on a simple meal of fish and vegetables as on a belly-buster. Surplus energy at night, especially alcohol and fat calories, is readily stored. This happens during sleep in particular, when everything's working at very slow rates.

Breakfast is probably the most important meal of the day. If you have a good one, it sets up your eating habits for the day and kick-starts your metabolism. This meal is essential and should never be missed. If you really find it difficult, work into it slowly.

Try just having some fruit salad with a bit of yoghurt if you're not a cook.

Lunch is a sustainer. Without it you'll perform badly later on in the day and feel tired and listless. Eat some kind of low GI grains, pasta, rice or cereal food with some meat, fish or poultry and a serving or two of vegetables or fruit.

Evening meals should be eaten by eight o'clock to allow at least partial digestion in the stomach to occur before sleep. Try to eat easily digestible food in the evening. One way to give your stomach a helping hand is to not mix starchy carbohydrates with high-protein foods in the same meal. The body utilizes protein at night to regenerate muscle tissue, so it's a good time to eat it. Also try to eat some kind of animal protein that is easy to digest (fish is excellent) and heaps of vegetables.

Rule 3

Be organized with the food you keep in the house and the food you order in restaurants.

Your ability to eat the right food at home starts when you go shopping, because what you buy is what you eat. Plan (at least when you're in the early stages of your fitness programme) what you are going to eat that week and stock up on it, so that when you open the fridge you'll find it easier to stay with the plan. It's easy to go off track when you open the fridge and are faced with junk food. If you keep an emergency stock of food, make that the good stuff too.

Same deal with restaurants, really. Don't pick restaurants that serve the wrong sorts of food. Make it easy for yourself. Find restaurants that will do as you ask. When you tell them to go easy on the oil or grill your fish rather than fry it make sure they do. In the United States you can go into the very best restaurants and they will steam your vegetables and grill your chicken without batting an eyelid if you ask them to. Try the same in England and insist on it. Punch the staff if you need to.

Rule 4

Keep a food diary, even if it's only in your head.

Keep a mental note of what you eat, or write it down. Then you can see when you go wrong and not do it again. Sometimes this helps in overcoming a specific habit that doesn't become apparent until you see it written down.

For instance, you might find that at 3 pm every day you feel tempted to eat something fattening. Do you pass the biscuit tin on the way to the bathroom? Are you not eating enough at lunchtime because you're too busy? Whatever the reason, by being aware of it you have a greater chance of overcoming it.

Eating correctly is food management. It doesn't happen by chance, but because you make it happen, and a diary will assist you in your mission.

Richard's clients (that poor down-trodden bunch) are asked to write a diary and some are sceptical about it because it seems a bit over the top. It might be if you had to do it for ever, but you don't. You only have do it until you're comfortable with your food routine and have organized it properly.

One client's entry under the midday meal was commonly 'Missed lunch, too busy.' The repercussions from this were that she felt tempted to eat biscuits mid-afternoon. In the end she overcame the lunch problem by making up her own at home and taking it to work with her. She didn't miss lunch after that because she didn't need to.

A diary need not take more than three or four minutes a day to fill out and it will help. Here's an example of how it could look:

Day: Monday Date: 17 June

Meal	Contents	Remarks
breakfast	yoghurt, chopped fruit, muesli, skimmed milk, 1 piece toast and fish spread	Bang on – didn't feel hungry till snack.
snack	piece of fruit	Only had a banana. Get cherries tomorrow – better.
lunch	pasta, salad, bread, fruit	Couldn't resist eating some bread. They put it on the table, so I ate it. Didn't really need it.
snack		Long meeting – missed my snack. Should have eaten it before I went in, really.
dinner	fish, steamed vegetables, fruit (2 pieces)	Back on track this evening. Feel better.

As you can see, the remarks column really helps. It gives you control. You make decisions. This is why we're born with a brain. Chimpanzees in zoos follow the dictates of others about what they should eat. We don't have to. Take control.

Rule 5

Maintain some balance in your attitude to food management. Don't panic.

This sounds a fairly unspecific rule, but it's probably the most important one and it's at the root of healthy eating. It means don't try to fit your life around the suggestions in this book, or indeed any book. Fit the book into your life. Everything is about balance.

Take the swing of the pendulum. If it swings a little to the left, it will swing a little to the right. If the swing is increased, it will increase both sides. If you mess up on one meal, it takes the equivalent of only a little swing to put it right by making a small adjustment. Don't give up. Don't go and buy a bag of choccies. Note the error and mend it.

Food intake is not really about management, it's about micro-management. Little movements either side of the path. Keep a sense of perspective.

Summary

These food rules should be tied in with the ideas behind the pyramid food system. They complement each other. Most of the information is self-explanatory. Once you understand you'll find it easy.

11
Eating Out in Restaurants

Eating out is a part of our lives and we can't ignore it. For some of us it accounts for the majority of what we eat, so it's important to take control.

The simplest solution is to go to which ever restaurant you like, eat what you want and negate the effects by especially diligent food and exercise routines over the next three to four days. Remember, no one gets fat from one meal. It takes a number of them to achieve that. Eating out once every three weeks is a viable option if you have the self-control to come back on line the following day.

The other scenario is that you eat out, albeit a work lunch, five times a week (maybe a third of your main meals). In this case, it won't work, because you're establishing a pattern which good meals and exercise cannot negate.

Eating too much and then going berserk on the treadmill the next day leads to tiredness, and endangers your health. Don't do it.

The best solution is to choose restaurants that offer healthy food and make selections that tie in with what you want to achieve. But if this is not possible, you have to practise damage limitation.

In many Indian restaurants, for example, the choice of low-fat foods is limited. So you end up making the best of a bad situation. If you can choose healthy restaurants most of the time, the odd curry – once every two or three weeks – isn't so damaging. Cooking varies from country to country and in some restaurants it is easier to eat healthily than it is in others.

Eating out – top tips

- Eat smaller portions of high GI foods and fatty foods. By trying even a spoonful of someone else's food, you can assuage your desire without having to order it yourself. If there's something you really want but shouldn't be eating, share it with someone else. Do this with puds in particular.

- Ask the waiter not to bring bread and butter to the table. If it's not there, it's not such a temptation.
- Ask the waiter if they can serve dressings and sauces separately. Then you can control how much you use, or skip them altogether if you want to.
- If you want your fish grilled instead of pan-fried, ask for it. It's your meal.
- Ask them to reduce the amounts of fattening items like cheese or butter that come with the dish.
- If you must have a fattening dish, ask for it as a starter portion. Take care to order something with it that will fill you up. If you eat small portions throughout the meal, you'll still be hungry at the end. Soup and plain pasta are good fillers.
- Serving sizes are just as relevant in restaurants as at home. Go to a restaurant knowing what you can eat in terms of servings. For example:
    one serving of meat, fish, poultry, etc.
    two servings of vegetables
    three servings of grains, rice, pasta, cereals, etc.
In this way, as long as you tie in the food with fat content and (if possible) GI value, you're much more likely to stay on track.

Let's now look at the restaurants in the high street, including fast-food outlets and see what's good.

The British café

Cafés rely on the griddle or deep-fat fryer to cook a lot of their food. Try to avoid items that are cooked in this way. Alternatives, though limited, include:

- baked beans on dry brown toast
- poached eggs on dry brown toast
- baked potato (high GI, though) and a low-fat filling like tuna and sweetcorn or chicken strips with peppers
- soup and dry brown bread or toast
- a wholemeal sandwich or roll with a salad and lean meat, fish or poultry filling
- fruit.

Avoid mayonnaise, coleslaw, butter, margarine and sugary sweets and confectionery.

Italian restaurants

Italian cooking uses a lot of olive oil. Although this is healthy in comparison to saturated fat, it's still fattening. Cheeses like mozzarella and Parmesan are also widely used. This is especially true of fast-food versions of Italian foods like pizza. Most of their traditional bread is refined with flour and ciabatta is made using large quantities of olive oil, which boosts its calorie content. So:

- Maximize on the excellent fresh salads available. Ask for dressing on the side or use lemon juice instead.
- Aim for tomato-based pasta sauces instead of the cream ones like carbonara, which sometimes has bacon with it as well. Limit or avoid the amount of Parmesan cheese you put on top of it. Ask the waiter to give you the spoon so you can add your own Parmesan.
- Pizzas: ask for less cheese on top. Stay away from pepperoni or chorizo sausage toppings, because they have a high fat content.
- Antipasti: these cold meat and vegetable starters are very oily. Keep away from them if you can.
- Pizza bases soaked in olive oil and garlic are not good news. Avoid them or, if you do eat one, be careful with the other choices you make.
- Start by filling up on a large healthy salad. It will make it easier to eat smaller portions of more fattening items on the menu later.
- Don't eat the bread and butter, since so much Italian food, like risotto, pasta and pizza, is carbohydrate-based.
- Visualize your pasta and pizza in servings from your grains, rice, cereals, etc. group. Eat that amount and no more.
- Avoid cream-based sweets like tiramisu or zabaglione, or just have a spoonful of someone else's. It's quite sexy if you're with a girl. If you're with a bloke – eat fruit on your own.

Indian restaurants

Indian food can be difficult. A lot of the meat and vegetable dishes are fried in ghee or butter. Ghee is butter made from buffalo milk and is very high in saturated fat. Indian restaurants use a lot of it, which affects the fat content badly in many of their dishes. If you eat them, it's a case of minimizing damage rather than going for healthy options. Here are some guidelines:

- Boiled rice should be chosen over the fried variety.
- Chapattis made with flour and water should be chosen over naan or paratha bread, to which fat is added.
- Stay away from cream-based curries like khorma dishes.
- Discard a proportion of the curry sauce from curry dishes. A lot of the fat content is in the sauce, and you always get too much anyway. Leave enough to make the dish palatable though.
- If you can't eat one poppadom without eating four, don't order them. They are deep-fat fried and highly fattening.
- Chicken tikka is comparatively low fat. This is a good option.
- Stay away from or minimize eating bhaji vegetable dishes (onion, mushroom and cauliflower). Again, they are deep-fat.
- If you usually drink lager with curries to cool down, drink cold mineral water instead. It's just as cooling and, unlike lager, doesn't have a GI figure higher than pure glucose.

Chinese restaurants

Chinese food is cooked in a wok or a deep-fat fryer. The wok cooks the food quickly, which means vitamins are less affected by it. However, Chinese food in general is a high-fat type, especially the dishes that are deep-fried in batter. Some suggestions are as follows:

- Make boiled rice (not fried rice or fried noodles) the base of your meal.
- Avoid dishes that include deep-fried batter.
- Meat and vegetable dishes are a good option.
- Chinese whole-fish dishes are sometimes baked in tin foil. This is another good option.
- Beware: duck skin contains large amounts of fat. Avoid it, or eat as little as possible.
- The same goes for pancake rolls.
- Sweet and sour sauce, hoisin sauce and black bean sauces contain a lot of sugar, so don't have too much.
- For dessert, choose the fruit on offer. Don't eat bananas in batter with treacle. If you must, have a mouthful of someone else's.

Japanese restaurants

Japanese food is mostly very healthy. There are lots of good options to choose from and it's very nutritious. Apart from one or two notable exceptions, I suggest you go for it.

- Raw fish on its own or with rice and seaweed is low in fat and high in carbohydrates and vitamin and mineral content. Eat it. It's called sashimi and it tastes great.
- The Japanese rice that is served with sushi has a high salt content. If you make your own you can lessen the amounts of salt without badly affecting the taste. In restaurants just go with the flow. (The price of Japanese food is going to stop you going too often anyway.)
- Stay away from, or eat small portions of, the tempura batter-fried dishes.
- Drink moderate amounts of the sake (rice wine). It's high on the GI and its alcohol content is higher than that of normal wine, making it calorie-loaded. A better choice is the green tea.
- The Japanese cook a lot of their vegetables on the griddle, but they use little oil so don't worry.
- Sweets are limited. They go for beautifully prepared fresh fruit, so that's a good option. Some restaurants serve a rather nasty dish called fried ice cream which is ice cream deep-fat fried in batter. Enough said.

Fast-food outlets

It's very difficult to give any tips about the type of food available from these places. There are healthy options in some of them, like salads, fruit juices, corn on the cob and fruit salads. If you go there for these types of dishes, great. Most people don't go for these things, however. (There are better places to buy them.) It's generally burgers, fries and milkshakes that people buy in fast-food outlets. Giving damage limitation tips on these items is difficult.

Look at the fat contents lists below for the most widely sold items from McDonald's, Kentucky Fried Chicken and Burger King and you'll see what I mean.

McDonald's

	Serving	Calories	Fat	Calories from Fat	% of Fat
hamburger in bun	102 g	255	9 g	81	31 %
quarter pounder	166 g	305	13 g	117	38 %
quarter pounder with cheese	194 g	510	28 g	252	49 %
French fries (small)	68 g	220	12g	108	49 %
chicken nuggets	6 pieces	270	15g	135	50 %

Burger King

	Serving	Calories	Fat	Calories from Fat	% of Fat
double burger sandwich with cheese	375 g	935	61 g	549	58 %
hamburger in bun	108 g	272	11 g	99	36 %

Kentucky Fried Chicken

	Serving	Calories	Fat	Calories from Fat	% of Fat
chicken wing	55 g	178	11.7 g	105.3	58 %
chicken thigh	104 g	294	19.7 g	177.3	60 %
chicken sandwich	166 g	482	27.3	245.7	50 %

(Adapted from *Introduction to Nutrition, Exercise and Health,* by Frank I. Katch and William D McArdle [Lea and Febiger, 1993])

Percentages of fat content range from about 30 per cent for a very basic item like a burger in a bun right up to 60 per cent for the more 'deluxe' version with cheese and bacon added.

If you eat regularly from outlets like these, you don't stand a chance. If they're your only option, eat enough to assuage your hunger until you can eat something better. Don't use such outlets regularly – once a month if you get caught out, and that's it. This might sound harsh, but sometimes it's better to tell it like it is. And that's how it is.

Serving sizes

All the suggestions given in this chapter have to be coupled with the food pyramid system. Have a idea before you go out how many servings from each group are available to you. Then bear in mind what a serving looks like in terms of size or quantity. For instance, a serving is:

- a slice of bread
- a slice of medium-sized pizza
- half a cup of cereal, rice, pasta or potatoes
- half a cup of most vegetables
- a small bowl of mixed salad
- a deck-of-cards-sized portion of meat, fish or poultry
- a cup of cooked beans
- one egg
- a small (25-gram/1-ounce) cube of cheese
- a cup of yoghurt or milk (skimmed).

If you tie this in with the top of the pyramid and limit or avoid fat, sweets and oil, you're getting there.

Summary

If you eat out:

- Choose as healthy a restaurant as is feasible.
- Know what servings you have available from the pyramid food groups for the meal and what a serving looks like.
- Make wise choices from the menu and micro-adjust dishes to suit your eating habits. You're paying for it.
- If you have to eat in a really bad restaurant, eat enough to assuage your hunger and then wait till you can eat something better elsewhere.

12
Recipes

Breakfast recipes

Orange nutmeg pan toast

Eat this breakfast after your morning aerobic work-out when your blood sugar levels are low and your glycogen stores need boosting.

    1 egg
    100 ml (4 fl oz) skimmed milk
    1 tsp grated orange rind
    ¼ tsp grated nutmeg
    8 pieces preferred low GI bread
    100 ml (4 fl oz) maple syrup
    1 tbsp icing sugar

Put the egg, milk, 2 tbsp water, the orange rind and nutmeg in a large shallow dish and whisk to combine. Place the bread slices in the egg mixture to coat one side, then immediately turn the bread. Let it stand for at least 10 minutes. Warm the syrup in a small saucepan. Preheat a non-stick griddle or a large non-stick frying pan over a medium heat. Brown both sides of the bread slices on the griddle or in the pan. Sprinkle the bread with a little icing sugar and serve with syrup. You can also serve with fruit (low GI like stoned cherries or sliced fresh peaches or apricots) or low-fat yoghurt, or both.

4 servings

Calories (per serving)	270
85 per cent carbohydrate	60 g
8 per cent protein	6 g
7 per cent fat	2 g
Low/medium GI	

Low-fat scrambled eggs with spinach

A satisfying breakfast containing all the major food groups but with low fat. Good to eat after a morning work-out with weights.

3 egg whites
1 egg yolk
1 piece preferred low GI bread
handful (preferably young) spinach
2 tbsp skimmed milk
1 tsp butter

Mix the egg whites, egg yolk, skimmed milk and butter in a saucepan. Cook over a low heat, stirring the mixture to prevent burning. Toast the bread. Plunge the spinach into boiling water till the leaves have collapsed (about 30 seconds), then remove and drain. Once the scrambled eggs are at the desired consistency, mix in the spinach and stir. Serve on the dry toast and season with pepper. (You can add roasted peppers for a mineral boost.)

1 serving

Calories	245
45 per cent carbohydrate	27 g
41 per cent protein	25 g
14 per cent fat	4 g
Low GI	

Porridge

Although porridge is a medium GI food, at breakfast this is not a problem, since your blood sugar levels will be low, especially if you've exercised aerobically for 20 minutes before breakfast.

2/3 cup porridge oats
2 cups water or low-fat milk
1/4 tsp salt (if desired)

Cook the porridge according to the packet instructions. You can boost the protein content by adding low-fat yoghurt or skimmed milk as desired. Fruit sweetens it without the calories of the sugary flavours. Try adding sliced stoned fruits (cherries, apricots, peaches, etc.), raisins or chopped banana. Flavour with 2 tsp honey, brown sugar, molasses or maple syrup.

1 serving

²/₃ cup pre-cooked porridge oats with ¹/₂ cup of low-fat milk:

Calories	285
60 per cent carbohydrate	44 g
25 per cent protein	17 g
15 per cent fat	5 g
Medium GI	

Prune-orange spread on toast

This is a good alternative to jams or marmalade which have very high sugar levels.

10 stoned prunes
100 ml (4 fl oz) orange juice
¹/₂ tsp pure vanilla extract
150 g (5¹/₂ oz) low-fat cottage cheese
6 slices cracked wheat bread (or preferred type)

Put the prunes, orange juice and vanilla extract in a small saucepan and cook, covered, over a medium heat for about 15 minutes or until the prunes are tender. Transfer the prunes and liquid to a food processor or blender and purée. Add the cottage cheese and process the mixture until smooth. Toast the bread and spread some of the prune mixture on each slice.

6 servings

Calories (per serving)	130
75 per cent carbohydrate	25 g
18 per cent protein	6 g
7 per cent fat	1 g
Low GI	

Wake-up shake

Good for a quick but nutritious breakfast.

1 stoned fruit (e.g. apricot, nectarine, peach)
200 ml (8 fl oz) low-fat yoghurt
4 tbsp orange juice
2 tbsp wheatgerm
2 ice-cubes

Place all the ingredients in a blender. Blend until thick and frothy.

1 serving

Calories	340
62 per cent carbohydrate	55 g
25 per cent protein	22 g
13 per cent fat	5 g
Low/medium GI	

Pasta

Pasta sauce base

To be used as a base for other pasta sauces.

2 tsp olive oil
1/2 cup finely chopped onions
2 garlic cloves, crushed
2 large red peppers (ribs and seeds removed), chopped
1/4 cup chicken broth
salt
ground pepper

Heat the olive oil in a large saucepan, over a medium heat. Add the onion, garlic and peppers. Cook for 3–5 minutes, until onion is translucent, stirring occasionally. Add the chicken broth; simmer for 4–5 minutes until vegetables are tender.

Mediterranean garden pasta

450 g (1 lb) spaghetti, fettuccini or linguine
pasta sauce base (see above)
1 cup chopped courgettes
1 can rinsed, drained cannellini beans
2 large ripe tomatoes, chopped
2 tbsp chopped fresh oregano or 1/2 tsp dried oregano
1/4 cup chopped fresh basil
1/4 cup white vinegar
grated Parmesan cheese (optional)

Cook pasta according to packet instructions. Drain. In a large saucepan, over medium heat, combine the pasta sauce base, courgettes, beans, tomatoes and oregano. Simmer for 5–10 minutes, or until the courgettes are tender. Just before serving, stir in the basil and vinegar. Serve in a large bowl and toss pasta in the sauce. Add a little Parmesan cheese if desired.

6 servings

Calories (per serving)	381
80 per cent carbohydrates	72g
15 per cent protein	14 g
5 per cent fat	4 g
Low/medium GI	

Pasta with tomato and mushroom sauce

1 large can (940 g/33.3 oz) plum tomatoes, undrained
1/2 cup chopped onion
2 garlic cloves, finely chopped
2 tsp fresh or dried basil
1/2 tsp crushed red pepper flakes
2 squirts olive oil cooking spray
2 cups sliced mushrooms
1/2 cup chopped green pepper
1 pack (450 g/1 lb) pasta, cooked and drained

In a medium saucepan, over a medium-high heat, combine the tomatoes, onion, garlic, basil and red pepper flakes. Bring to the boil. Reduce the heat to low; cover and simmer for 10–20 minutes, or until the liquid is reduced by half. Cool slightly. Meanwhile spray a non-stick frying pan with olive oil and place over a medium-high heat. Add the mushrooms and green pepper. Cook, stirring frequently, for 5 minutes, until cooked but still crisp. Set aside. Purée the tomato sauce to the desired consistency. Then add to the mushrooms and peppers in the saucepan. Heat and pour on to the cooked pasta.

8 servings

Calories (per serving)	247
81 per cent carbohydrates	50 g
15 per cent protein	9 g
4 per cent fat	1 g
Low/medium GI	

Seafood noodles with peas and watercress

450 g (1 lb) medium egg noodles or bow-tie pasta (farfalle)
350 g (12 oz) medium shelled prawns
1 tbsp seafood seasoning
pasta sauce base (see page 99)
250 g (9 oz) frozen or canned artichoke hearts or 2 cups fresh mushrooms
1 cup fresh or frozen peas
1 bunch watercress (tough stems removed)

Cook the noodles or pasta according to instructions; drain. Mix the prawns with the seafood seasoning in large saucepan, over a medium heat. Mix in the pasta sauce base, prawns, artichoke hearts or mushrooms, peas and watercress. Simmer for 3 minutes, or until the prawns turn opaque, stirring occasionally. Serve in a large bowl, tossing the cooked noodles in the hot sauce.

6 servings

Calories (per serving)	412
65 per cent carbohydrates	66 g
22 per cent protein	23 g
13 per cent fat	6 g
Low-GI	

Pasta and beans

This is a very high carbohydrate dish and the beans are very low GI. Beans are also high in protein. A good meal to have a couple of hours before a long aerobic work-out.

225 g (8 oz) uncooked pasta
350-g (12-oz) jar salsa
325-g (11-oz) can corn
425-g (15-oz) can white or pinto beans, drained and rinsed
3 tbsp grated low-fat Cheddar cheese
2 tbsp chopped coriander

Cook the pasta according to the instructions on the package. Drain well. Combine the salsa, corn and beans in a large pot and heat thoroughly. Add the pasta and mix well. Sprinkle the cheese on top and garnish with coriander.

5 servings

Calories (per serving)	470
50 per cent carbohydrates	60 g
46 per cent protein	54 g
4 per cent fat	2 g
Low GI	

Sesame pasta with broccoli

This is a dish high in minerals and carbohydrates, but low in fat. It's also simple and quick to cook.

225 g (8 oz) pasta
2 cups fresh chopped broccoli
1/4 cup tahini (sesame butter)
1 tsp olive oil
1 small scallion
1/2 cup chopped celery
cayenne pepper to taste

Cook the pasta according to the packet instructions and drain. While the pasta is cooking, steam the broccoli until tender but still crisp. Reserve a little of the cooking liquid (see below). Fry the celery and scallion in the olive oil until cooked. Mix tahini with the drained pasta then add celery, scallion and broccoli. Stir well. If the pasta is dry, add a small amount of the broccoli cooking liquid to moisten.

2 servings

Calories (per serving)	350
60 per cent carbohydrates	50 g
15 per cent protein	15 g
25 per cent fat	10 g
Low GI	

Soups

Fish and broccoli soup

Followed by salad, this makes a good lunch. If you want it to be more sustaining, add some noodles or low GI rice (Basmati).

1 cup chicken broth (any type, home-made or from a cube)
225 g (8 oz) white fish cut into 2.5-cm (1-inch) cubes
1 cup fresh broccoli
1/4 tsp sesame oil

Heat the chicken broth. Add the fish, chopped broccoli and sesame oil. Bring to the boil, then turn down the heat. Simmer for about 5 minutes, or until the broccoli is tender and the fish translucent.

1 serving

Calories	200
25 per cent carbohydrates	15 g
70 per cent protein	33 g
5 per cent fat	2 g
Low/medium GI	

Leek and potato soup

This soup is low in sodium and fat but very filling; a cupful is a good snack.

4 leeks
2 potatoes, peeled and quartered
110 g (4 oz) celery, thinly sliced
1 litre (1 3/4 pints) low-sodium chicken stock
440 ml (16 fl oz) skimmed milk
1 tbsp chopped fresh parsley
white pepper

Cut off the root ends and green tops from the leeks. Halve the leeks length-wise, separate the layers and wash them thoroughly. Cut them into 2.5-cm (1-inch) pieces. In a large saucepan, combine the leeks, potatoes, celery and stock. Bring to the boil, skimming off the oil. Reduce the heat and simmer, uncovered, for about 40 minutes or until the vegetables are tender. Cool the soup briefly, then purée in a blender or food processor or mash to a coarse purée by hand. Add the milk and reheat the soup until just heated through; do not boil. Ladle into bowls or cups and sprinkle with parsley and pepper.

4 servings

Calories (per serving)	120
74 per cent carbohydrates	23 g
25 per cent protein	8 g
1 per cent fat	trace
Medium GI	

Cream of green pea soup

High in protein, minerals and fibre, this soup is also low GI.

    heart of a cos lettuce
    450 g (1 lb) fresh peas (frozen will do)
    25 g (1 oz) butter
    570 ml (1 pint) water
    1.1 litres (2 pints) skimmed milk
    seasoning
    75 g (3 oz) tofu

Chop the lettuce heart and cook with the peas and the butter in a pan for a few moments before adding the water. Let the mixture simmer for 15 minutes, then allow to cool. Add the milk, seasoning and tofu. Liquidize the soup to a thin purée. Reheat gently and serve. (To add more protein, add some chopped lean ham.)

6 servings

Calories (per serving)	160
45 per cent carbohydrate	18 g
30 per cent protein	12 g
25 per cent fat	5 g
Low GI	

Carrot and ginger soup

This is a good soup to bring low blood sugar levels back up after a hard work-out. Eaten with a pasta dish it is even better, since it will restore glycogen levels.

    10 g (1/2 oz) butter or 1/2 tbsp olive oil
    700 g (1 1/2 lb) carrots, washed, trimmed and chopped
    1 small onion, chopped
    1/2 tbsp ginger root
    1.75 litres (3 pints) vegetable or chicken stock
    1 tbsp raspberry vinegar
    salt and pepper

Heat the butter or oil in a large saucepan, add the carrots, ginger and onion and cook for 2 minutes. Add the stock and simmer for a further 10 minutes. Liquidize the vegetables to a purée, adding stock till the desired consistency is reached. Finally, stir in the raspberry vinegar and season with salt and pepper.

6 servings

Calories (per serving)	60
49 per cent carbohydrate	6 g
6 per cent protein	1 g
45 per cent fat	3 g
High GI	

Sandwich fillings

Lower GI bread options are:

- oat bran bread
- barley kernel bread
- rye kernel bread
- rye bagel
- pumpernickel and pumpernickel bagel
- wholemeal pitta bread
- bulgar wheat bread
- 50 per cent kibbled wheat-grain bread

Try to use these types with the following recipes, as they will help give you long-term energy and help reduce body-fat levels. Stay away from French baguettes (very fattening). In addition, cut out the butter or spreads. The normal calorific value of butter for bread is 90 calories. Some of the recipe suggestions include soft cheeses, which should contain enough fat for flavour. Use fresh herbs for added flavour.

Mozzarella and basil sandwich

    buffalo mozzarella
    basil leaves
    a beef tomato

Lay thin slices of mozzarella on the bread, followed by thin slices of beef tomato. Finally, cover with the basil leaves.

Ham and coleslaw sandwich

    thin sliced ham (without fat)
    coleslaw (made with low-fat mayonnaise)
    mustard cress

Pile on to bread, without butter.

Pastrami and grilled vegetables

    pastrami
    courgettes
    aubergines
    peppers
    olive oil spray
    salt and pepper
    oak-leaf lettuce

Thinly slice the vegetables and spray with olive oil. Grill until they are just beginning to char. Pile ingredients onto barley-kernel bread. Season with salt and pepper, spray on a little more olive oil and eat.

Lime chicken on bread

    roast chicken off the bone
    low-fat yoghurt or light mayonnaise
    yellow peppers, finely chopped
    spring onion, finely chopped
    lime juice
    thyme
    black pepper

Chop the chicken into small pieces and mix with all the other ingredients.

Tuna and rocket

    tuna fish in brine
    low-fat yoghurt or light mayonnaise
    finely chopped red or green peppers
    rocket leaves
    salt and pepper

Drain the tuna and mix with the yoghurt or mayonnaise. Do not use butter. Create a bed of rocket on a toasted pumpernickel bagel and then spoon on the mixture.

Lamb in pitta bread

The chick-peas in this recipe provide cholesterol-lowering fibre as well as low GI, carbohydrate and usable protein.

8 wholemeal pittas
225 g (8 oz) lean minced lamb
35 g (1¹/₂ oz) chopped onion
2¹/₂ sweet green peppers
2 crushed garlic cloves
175-g (6-oz) can tomatoes
175-g (6-oz) can chick-peas
35 g (1¹/₂ oz) black olives, chopped
1¹/₂ tsp chopped fresh rosemary
¹/₄ tsp cinnamon
225 ml (8 fl oz) plain low-fat yoghurt
4 tbsp chopped fresh mint
¹/₄ tsp salt
¹/₄ tsp ground pepper
25 g (1 oz) feta cheese, crumbed

Preheat the oven to 150°C/300°F/Gas Mark 2. Stack the pittas, wrap them in foil and set aside. In a medium-sized non-stick frying-pan, brown the lamb, onion, pepper and garlic over a medium-high heat. Spoon into a strainer to drain the fat and return to pan. Add the tomatoes and their liquid, the chick-peas, olives, rosemary and cinnamon, stirring and mashing the chick-peas and tomatoes with a spoon, and cook until heated through. Meanwhile, heat the pittas in the oven. Combine the yoghurt, mint, salt and pepper in a small bowl. Add the cheese to the frying pan and heat until the cheese melts. Cut a small slice from the top of each pitta. Spoon the lamb mixture into the pittas and top with the yoghurt mixture.

4 servings

Calories (per serving)	500
52 per cent carbohydrate	65 g
29 per cent protein	36 g
19 per cent fat	12 g
Low/medium GI	

Tabbouleh

Whole-grain foods like this contain more vitamins and fibre than refined versions. They are also lower GI, providing long-term energy without adversely affecting your blood sugar levels.

170 g (6 oz) burghul
50 g (2 oz) fresh chopped parsley
40 g (1½ oz fresh chopped mint
50 g (2 oz) spring onions (green and white parts), finely chopped
1 tbsp olive oil
2 tbsp lemon juice
½ tsp salt
2 medium tomatoes, chopped
a small head cos lettuce

Bring 425 ml (16 fl oz) of water to the boil in a small saucepan. Place the burghul in a large bowl and pour the boiling water over it. Let it stand for at least 2 hours. Then drain the burghul well in a strainer, pressing out the excess water. Return the burghul to the bowl, add the remaining ingredients, except the lettuce, and mix well. To serve, line a platter or salad bowl with lettuce leaves and pile the burghul on top.

4 servings

Calories (per serving)	195
64 per cent carbohydrate	32 g
16 per cent protein	8 g
20 per cent fat	4½ g
Low GI	

Tofu hummus with pitta crisps

Dips made from cheese or soured cream are rich in calcium, but can be very high in saturated fat. This version of hummus is made with tofu, sesame seeds and broccoli, which are amongst the best non-dairy sources of dietary calcium.

350 g (12 oz) firm tofu, cubed
175 g (6 oz) cooked or canned chick-peas, drained
3 tbsp lemon juice
1 tbsp tahini (sesame paste)
1 garlic clove, crushed
2 tbsp chopped fresh dill
6 small pitta breads
1 orange-fleshed sweet potato, boiled, cooled and peeled
¼ tsp salt
ground pepper
1½ tsp sesame seeds
100 g (4 oz) broccoli florets, blanched and cooled

Place the tofu in a food processor or blender with the chick-peas, lemon juice, tahini and garlic and process until smooth. Transfer the mixture to a serving bowl, stir in the dill, cover and refrigerate.

Preheat the oven to 180°C/350°F/Gas Mark 4. Split the pitta breads and cut each piece into quarters. Spread the pieces on a baking sheet and toast them for 10 minutes, or until lightly browned round the edges. Meanwhile, cut the sweet potato length-ways into four sticks. To serve, season the hummus with the salt and pepper to taste. Divide on to six plates and sprinkle each portion with some of the sesame seeds. Arrange the broccoli florets, sweet-potato sticks and pitta triangles round the hummus and serve.

6 servings

Calories (per serving)	235
60 per cent carbohydrate	36 g
20 per cent protein	12 g
20 per cent fat	5 g
Low/medium GI	

Brown rice and vegetable risotto

This version has half the fat of a normal risotto dish. Cheese amounts are also lower.

    25 g (1 oz) margarine
    90-g (3½-oz) courgette, julienned
    100-g (4-oz) red pepper, sliced thinly
    225 g (8 oz) broccoli florets
    ½ tsp dried oregano
    ½ tsp black pepper
    350 ml (12 fl oz) low-sodium chicken stock
    150 g (5 oz) spring onions, chopped
    185 g (6½ oz) brown rice
    4 tbsp grated Parmesan cheese
    4 tbsp chopped parsley

Melt half the margarine in a large non-stick frying-pan over a medium-high heat. Add the courgettes, peppers and broccoli and cook, stirring frequently, for 2 minutes, or until well coated with margarine. Add half the oregano, half of the pepper and 4 tbsp of stock, cover and cook for a further 2 minutes. Stir in the onions. Put the vegetables in a bowl and cover loosely to keep warm.

Melt the remaining margarine in the pan over a medium-high heat and sauté the rice for 2 minutes. Add 175 ml (6 fl oz) water and the remaining stock, oregano and pepper. Cover and reduce the heat to medium-low and simmer for 45 minutes, or until the rice is tender and most of the liquid is absorbed. Stir in the vegetables, Parmesan and parsley, and cook, stirring, over a medium-high heat for one minute or until heated through.

4 servings

Calories (per serving)	330
62 per cent carbohydrate	53 g
12 per cent protein	10 g
26 per cent fat	10 g
Medium GI	

Desserts

Blackcurrant poached pears

This is a low GI and low-fat sweet and is attractive enough to serve when entertaining.

2 firm dessert pears
225-g (8-oz) can unsweetened blackcurrants in own juice
1 glass red wine
1 tbsp fructose sugar
2 tbsp low-fat fromage frais

Peel the pears, leaving the stems intact. Put the blackcurrant juice, wine, water and sugar in a saucepan and heat slowly. Place the pears in this mixture so they are covered and cook for 20 minutes, until cooked but firm. Take out the pears and chill. Reduce the remaining liquid by half and chill as well. Serve in a bowl with blackcurrants and chilled reserved liquid with a tablespoon of fromage frais.

2 servings
Low GI

Baked apples

  2 medium cooking apples
  50 g (2 oz) raisins
  25 g (1 oz) chopped dates
  2 tbsp honey
  2 tbsp low-fat frozen yoghurt

Preheat the oven to 190°C/375°F/Gas Mark 5. Core the apples and score a line around the circumference of each with a sharp knife. Stuff the apples with raisins and dates and pour the honey over the top. Bake for 25 minutes (or until the apples are soft). Serve with one tablespoon of frozen yoghurt per person.

2 servings
Low/medium GI

GI Joe fruit salad

A delicious low-fat combination of low GI fruits packed with vitamins. Also delicious for breakfast.

  1/2 cup cherries
  1/2 cup strawberries
  1 grapefruit
  1 peach
  2 apricots
  1 pear
  juice of 1 lemon
  1 tbsp fructose sugar

Wash and chop up all the fruits into bite-size pieces, leaving the skins on for fibre (remembering, of course, to peel the grapefruit!). Mix together with the lemon juice and fructose. Chill and serve with a little low-fat yoghurt if desired.

3 servings
Low GI

Fruit jelly with strawberry sauce

A great low-fat alternative to trifle. Can be made in individual ramekins for a dinner party if you're feeling fancy!

  2 1/2 tsp gelatine
  100 ml (4 fl oz) fresh orange juice

275 ml (10 fl oz) grapefruit juice
4 tbsp unsweetened apple juice
1½ tbsp fresh lime juice
3 tbsp fructose sugar
1 melon, halved
225 g (8 oz) strawberries
1 kiwi fruit, peeled and thinly sliced

Dissolve gelatine in 3 tablespoons of water and leave for 5 minutes. Combine all the juices with 2 tablespoons of the sugar in a pan, reserving half a teaspoon of the fresh lime. Bring to the boil and remove immediately from heat. Stir in the gelatine mixture and chill for 30 minutes until syrupy and then keep at room temperature. Chop the melon into small pieces and place in large dessert bowl. Cover with half the jelly mixture and leave to set. Slice half the strawberries and layer them (attractively if you have time) on top of the set jelly and melon, cover with the rest of the jelly mixture and leave to set. To make the sauce, purée the remaining strawberries with the remaining lime juice and sugar and chill.

6 servings
Low/medium GI

Fruit fool

This is low-fat dessert containing low GI fruit. Another breakfast alternative or snack.

2 egg-whites
1 cup ripe strawberries
1 cup ripe raspberries
1 cup ripe cherries, stoned
175 g (6 oz) natural low-fat yoghurt
3 tbsp wheatgerm or muesli (optional)

Liquidize the fruit. Beat the egg-whites until stiff. Fold the yoghurt into the egg-whites. Fold this mixture carefully into the liquidized fruits. Chill. Serve in tall glasses topped with a tablespoon of wheatgerm or muesli if desired.

3 servings
Low GI

13
Preparing to Exercise

We've talked a lot in previous chapters about food, but that's really only part of the equation for the new you. Exercise is the other bit that makes it happen. It's the big one. Losing weight makes you thinner, but it doesn't necessarily make you healthier. (For example, look at a certain former Chancellor of the Exchequer who lost a lot of weight and still looks awful.)

Fitness assessment

Before you start training it's important that you assess your present level of fitness, and find out your body statistics. No matter how fat you are, you can begin to change for the better.

Once you know exactly how bad the situation is, you can begin to plan the programme that will drag you out of your current state and into fitness.

Medical check-up

Before you start a training programme go and see your doctor. He will be delighted to assess your fitness, because doctors get paid for people on their list whether they get sick or not – and fit people are profitable people to the medical profession. Your doctor will also tell you whether you are fit enough to start hurting yourself.

A medical check-up is especially relevant if any of the following apply to you:

- You are over 30 and have led a sedentary life for the last three months.
- You have been a heart patient.
- You are a stroke victim.
- You are diabetic.
- You have had an asthmatic condition.
- You have high blood pressure.
- You are clinically obese.
- You have muscular or skeletal problems.

Body statistics

The next step is to get your basic statistics down on paper, so find a cloth tape-measure and fill in the following chart. If you don't want to write in the book (thus ruining its value as a first edition), photocopy the page or write out the list on a piece of paper.

---

chest/bust (over nipple line)

biceps (relaxed state; widest point)
   right
   left

waist (over navel)

hips (at widest point)

top of thigh
   right
   left

calf (at widest point)
   right
   left

weight

resting pulse (beats per minute – measure first thing in the
   morning and average out over four days)

Body-fat percentage

The next thing you need to measure is body fat. Rather than use body-fat callipers, which are not widely available to most people, Richard often uses a method pioneered by Dr Michael Eades from his book *Thin So Fast*. Although not absolutely accurate, it is within permissible limits (body fat calliper accuracy is not 100 per cent accurate either).

Method

For women:

1. Measure your hips at their widest point and your waist over the navel. Do the measurement – in inches – two or three times, over several days, then take the averages. Use the worksheet below to record the measurements.

2. Measure your height in inches while barefoot. Record this measurement.

3. Turn to the table on page 120 and find the measurements. Now look at the right column and note on the worksheet the accompanying constant.

4. Add constants A and B together, then subtract constant C. Round off the figure to the nearest whole number. That figure is your approximate body-fat percentage.

average hip measurement	.... inches	constant A ....
average waist measurement	.... inches	constant B ....
height	.... inches	constant C ....
constant A + constant B		= ....
minus constant C		= ....
body-fat percentage		= .... %

For men

1. Measure – in inches – your waist over your navel and the wrist of your dominant hand (measure where your wrist bends). Do the measurements two or three times over a few days, then take the averages. Record these average measurements on the worksheet below.

2. Subtract your wrist measurement from your waist measurement and find the resulting value at the top of the table on page 118. Now, in the column on the left-hand side of the table, find your weight (in pounds). Look directly across from your weight and down from your waist/wrist measurement. The figure at the point where they intersect is your approximate body-fat percentage.

(a) average waist measurement	....
(b) average wrist measurement	....
(c) weight	.... lb
a – b	= ....

Find this figure (the remainder) at the top of the table on page 118, and (c) in the left-hand column and see where the two lines intersect.

body-fat percentage = ... %

Calculating body-fat weight and lean body weight

Now you know your body-fat percentage, you can find:

- the weight of your body-fat
- The weight of your lean body mass

To find your body-fat weight, multiply your weight in pounds by your body-fat percentage, then divide by 100. For example:

$$180 \text{ lb} \times 18 \text{ \% body fat} = 3240$$
$$3240 \div 100 = 32.4 \text{ lb body-fat weight}$$

To find your lean body mass (or lean muscle-mass weight) subtract your body-fat weight from your total body weight. For example:

$$180 \text{ lb} - 32.4 \text{ lb} = 147.6 \text{ lb lean body mass}$$

If you know your total weight, your body-fat percentage and your lean body mass, you can monitor the effect of your training programme more accurately. When you jump on the scales to see how much weight you have lost, you should want to know where that weight came from. Now you can answer that question.

So, as part of your body statistics list, you should record:

- your total body weight ....
- your body-fat percentage ....
- your body-fat weight ....

This will enable you to make comparisons later.

Fitness tests

There are various tests you can do to assess how fit you are so that you can choose the right intensity of aerobic exercise and a suitable strength training programme to start with. The tests will also show how flexible you are. Let's begin with the aerobic aspect.

Aerobic step test

Aerobic exercise can be divided into levels, or zones, of intensity. (This is covered on pages 128–136.) To decide which one is suitable, here is a simple test that you can do at home. You will need:

- a step 30 to 35 cm (about a foot) high
- appropriate loose clothing
- a watch with a second hand.

Practise performing the step test so that you can complete two 'up, up, down, down' cycles in 5 seconds. A friend can help by calling out the times.

Now step up and down for exactly three minutes. When you have stopped, sit down and rest for 30 seconds. Find your pulse. Count the number of beats for the next 30 seconds. Compare the result with the chart below:

Age:	20–29	30–39	40–49	50+	Rating
Men					
Number of beats	34–36	35–38	37–39	37–40	Excellent
	37–40	39–41	40–42	41–43	Good
	41–42	42–43	43–44	44–45	Average
	43–47	44–47	45–49	46–49	Fair
	48–59	48–59	50–60	50–62	Poor
Women					
Number of beats	39–42	39–42	41–43	41–44	Excellent
	43–44	43–45	44–45	45–47	Good
	45–46	46–47	46–47	48–49	Average
	47–52	48–53	48–54	50–55	Fair
	53–66	54–66	55–67	56–66	Poor

The following recommendations apply whether you are male or female, and whatever age you are.

- If your result is 'good' or 'excellent', you should be comfortable starting in Zone 2 (i.e. at 70 to 85 per cent of your Max HR).
- If your result is 'average', spend the first week or so of training in Zone 1 and then gradually move up to Zone 2 over the following week or when you feel up to it. Do not over-exert yourself.
- If your result is 'fair' or 'poor', you should exercise in Zone 1. Move to Zone 2 by slow stages and then only if it suits you. Some people find Zone 1 suits their purpose fine, either because of their age or because they like going for long walks. The reason is not important. It is an effective zone if the exercise is done for the prescribed amount of time.

Strength tests

The following tests will allow you to determine the best level for you to start your strength-training exercise, so you can select

Body-fat calculations: men

waist–wrist in inches / weight in lb	26.0	26.5	27.0	27.5	28.0	28.5	29.0	29.5	30.0	30.5	31.0	31.5	32.0	32.5	33.0	33.5	34.0	34.5	35.0	35.5	36.0
120	20	20	23	25	27	29	31	33	35	41	39	41	43	45	47	49	50	52	54		
125	19	19	22	24	26	28	30	32	33	39	37	39	41	43	45	46	48	50	52	54	
130	18	18	21	23	25	27	28	30	32	37	36	37	39	41	43	44	46	48	50	52	53
135	17	17	20	22	24	26	27	29	31	36	34	36	38	39	41	43	44	46	48	50	51
140	16	16	19	21	23	24	26	28	29	34	33	34	36	38	39	41	43	44	46	48	49
145	15	15	19	20	22	23	25	27	28	33	31	33	35	36	38	39	41	43	44	46	47
150	15	15	18	19	21	23	24	26	27	32	30	32	33	35	36	38	40	41	43	44	46
155	14	14	17	19	20	22	23	25	26	31	29	31	32	34	35	37	38	40	41	43	44
160	14	14	16	18	19	21	22	24	25	30	28	30	31	33	34	35	37	38	40	41	43
165	13	13	15	17	19	20	22	23	24	29	27	29	30	31	33	34	36	37	38	40	41
170	13	13	15	17	18	19	21	22	24	28	26	28	29	30	32	33	34	36	37	39	40
175	12	12	14	16	17	19	20	21	23	27	25	27	28	29	31	32	33	35	36	37	39
180	12	12	14	16	17	18	19	21	22	26	25	26	27	28	30	31	32	34	35	36	37
185	11	11	13	15	16	18	19	20	21	25	24	25	26	28	29	30	31	33	34	35	36
190	11	11	13	15	16	17	18	19	21	24	23	24	26	27	28	29	30	32	33	34	35
195	11	11	12	14	15	16	18	19	20	24	22	24	25	26	27	28	30	31	32	33	34
200	10	10	12	14	15	16	17	18	19	23	22	23	24	25	26	28	29	30	31	32	33
205	10	10	12	13	14	15	17	18	19	22	21	22	23	25	26	27	28	29	30	31	32
210	9	9	11	13	14	15	16	17	18	22	21	22	23	24	25	26	27	28	29	30	32
215	9	9	11	12	13	15	16	17	18	21	20	21	22	23	24	25	26	28	29	30	31
220	9	9	11	12	13	14	15	16	17	20	19	20	22	23	24	25	26	27	28	29	30
225	9	9	10	12	13	14	15	16	17	20	19	20	21	22	23	24	25	26	27	28	29
230	8	8	10	11	12	13	14	15	16	19	18	19	20	21	22	23	24	25	26	27	28
235	8	8	10	11	12	13	14	15	16	19	18	19	20	21	22	23	24	25	26	27	28
240	8	8	9	11	12	13	14	15	16	18	17	18	19	20	21	22	23	24	25	26	27
245	8	7	9	10	11	12	13	14	15	18	17	18	19	20	21	22	23	24	25	26	27
250	7	7	9	10	11	12	13	14	15	18	17	18	18	19	20	21	22	23	24	25	26
255	7	7	9	10	11	12	13	14	14	17	16	17	18	19	20	21	22	23	24	24	25
260	7	7	8	10	10	11	12	13	14	17	16	17	18	19	19	20	21	22	23	24	25
265	7	7	8	9	10	11	12	13	14	16	15	16	17	18	19	20	21	22	22	23	24
270	7	6	8	9	10	11	12	13	13	16	15	16	17	18	19	19	20	21	22	23	24
275	6	6	8	9	10	11	11	12	13	16	15	16	16	17	18	19	20	21	22	22	23
280	6	6	8	9	9	10	11	12	13	15	14	15	16	17	18	19	19	20	21	22	23
285	6	6	7	8	9	10	11	12	12	15	14	15	16	17	17	18	19	20	21	21	22
290	6	6	7	8	9	10	11	11	12	15	14	15	15	16	17	18	19	19	20	21	22
295	6	6	7	8	9	10	10	11	12	14	14	14	15	16	17	17	18	19	20	21	21
300	5	5	6	8	9	9	10	11	12	14	13	14	15	16	16	17	18	19	19	20	21

37.5	38.0	38.5	39.0	39.5	40.0	40.5	41.0	41.5	42.0	42.5	43.0	43.5	44.0	44.5	45.0	45.5	46.0	46.5	47.0	47.5	48.0	48.5	49.0
54																							
52	54	55																					
50	52	53	55																				
49	50	52	53	55																			
47	48	50	51	53	54																		
45	47	48	50	51	52	54	55																
44	45	47	48	49	51	52	54	55															
43	44	45	47	48	49	51	52	53	55														
41	43	44	45	47	48	49	50	52	53	54													
40	41	43	44	45	46	48	49	50	51	53	54	55											
39	40	41	43	44	45	46	48	49	50	51	52	54	55										
38	39	40	41	43	44	45	46	47	49	50	51	52	53	55									
37	38	39	40	41	43	44	45	46	47	48	50	51	52	53	54	55							
36	37	38	39	40	41	43	44	45	46	47	48	49	51	52	53	54	55						
35	36	37	38	39	40	42	43	44	45	46	47	48	49	50	51	53	54	55					
34	35	36	37	38	39	40	42	43	44	45	46	47	48	49	50	51	52	53	54	55			
33	34	35	36	37	38	39	41	42	43	44	45	46	47	48	49	50	51	52	53	54	55		
32	33	34	35	36	37	38	40	41	42	43	44	45	46	47	48	49	50	51	52	53	54	55	
32	33	34	35	36	37	38	39	40	41	42	44	44	45	46	47	48	49	50	51	52	53	54	55
31	32	33	34	35	36	37	38	39	40	41	42	43	44	45	46	47	48	49	50	51	51	52	53
30	31	32	33	34	35	36	37	38	39	40	41	42	43	44	45	46	46	47	48	49	50	51	52
29	30	31	32	33	34	35	36	37	38	39	40	41	42	43	44	44	45	46	47	48	49	50	51
29	30	31	31	32	33	34	35	36	37	38	39	40	41	42	43	44	44	45	46	47	48	49	50
28	29	30	31	32	33	34	34	35	36	37	38	39	40	41	42	43	44	44	45	46	47	48	49
27	28	29	30	31	32	33	34	35	35	36	37	38	39	40	41	42	43	43	44	45	46	47	48
27	28	29	29	30	31	32	33	34	35	36	36	37	38	39	40	41	42	43	43	44	45	46	47
26	27	28	29	30	31	31	32	33	34	35	36	37	37	38	39	40	41	42	43	43	44	45	46
26	27	27	28	29	30	31	32	32	33	34	35	36	37	38	38	39	40	41	42	43	43	44	45
25	26	27	28	29	29	30	31	32	33	33	34	35	36	37	38	38	39	40	41	42	43	43	44
25	26	26	27	28	29	30	30	31	32	33	34	34	35	36	37	38	39	39	40	41	42	43	43
24	25	26	27	27	28	29	30	31	31	32	33	34	35	35	36	37	38	39	39	40	41	42	43
24	25	25	26	27	28	28	29	30	31	32	32	33	34	35	36	36	37	38	39	39	40	41	42
23	24	25	26	26	27	28	29	29	30	31	32	33	33	34	35	36	36	37	38	39	39	40	41

Body-fat calculations: women

Hips		Abdomen		Height	
Inches	Constant	Inches	Constant	Inches	Constant
A		B		C	
30.0	33.48	20.0	14.22	55.0	33.52
30.5	33.83	20.5	14.40	55.5	33.67
31.0	34.87	21.0	14.93	56.0	34.13
31.5	35.22	21.5	15.11	56.5	34.28
32.0	36.27	22.0	15.64	57.0	34.74
32.5	36.62	22.5	15.82	57.5	34.89
33.0	37.67	23.0	16.35	58.0	35.35
33.5	38.02	23.5	16.53	58.5	35.50
34.0	39.06	24.0	17.06	59.0	35.96
34.5	39.41	24.5	17.24	59.5	36.11
35.0	40.46	25.0	17.78	60.0	36.57
35.5	40.81	25.5	17.96	60.5	36.72
36.0	41.86	26.0	18.49	61.0	37.18
36.5	42.21	26.5	18.67	61.5	37.33
37.0	43.25	27.0	19.20	62.0	37.79
37.5	43.60	27.5	19.38	62.5	37.94
38.0	44.65	28.0	19.91	63.0	38.40
38.5	45.32	28.5	20.27	63.5	38.70
39.0	46.05	29.0	20.62	64.0	39.01
39.5	46.40	29.5	20.80	64.5	39.16
40.0	47.44	30.0	21.33	65.0	39.62
40.5	47.79	30.5	21.51	65.5	39.77
41.0	48.84	31.0	22.04	66.0	40.23
41.5	49.19	31.5	22.22	66.5	40.38
42.0	50.24	32.0	22.75	67.0	40.84
42.5	50.59	32.5	22.93	67.5	40.99
43.0	51.64	33.0	23.46	68.0	41.45
43.5	51.99	33.5	23.64	68.5	41.60
44.0	53.03	34.0	24.18	69.0	42.06
44.5	53.41	34.5	24.36	69.5	42.21

Hips		Abdomen		Height	
Inches	Constant	Inches	Constant	Inches	Constant
A		B		C	
45.0	54.53	35.0	24.89	70.0	42.67
45.5	54.86	35.5	26.07	70.5	42.82
46.0	55.83	36.0	25.60	71.0	43.43
46.5	56.18	36.5	25.78	71.5	43.82
47.0	57.22	37.0	26.31	72.0	43.89
47.5	57.57	37.5	26.49	72.5	44.04
48.0	58.62	38.0	27.02	73.0	44.50
48.5	58.97	38.5	27.20	73.5	44.65
49.0	60.02	39.0	27.73	74.0	45.11
49.5	60.37	39.5	27.91	74.5	45.26
50.0	61.42	40.0	28.44	75.0	45.72
50.5	61.77	40.5	28.62	75.5	45.87
51.0	62.81	41.0	29.15	76.0	46.32
51.5	63.16	41.5	29.33		
52.0	64.21	42.0	29.87		
52.5	64.56	42.5	30.05		
53.0	65.61	43.0	30.58		
53.5	65.96	43.5	30.76		
54.0	67.00	44.0	31.29		
54.5	67.35	44.5	31.47		
55.0	68.40	45.0	32.00		
55.5	68.75	45.5	32.18		
56.0	69.80	46.0	32.71		
56.5	70.15	46.5	32.89		
57.0	71.19	47.0	33.42		
57.5	71.54	47.5	33.60		
58.0	72.59	48.0	34.13		
58.5	72.94	48.5	34.31		
59.0	73.99	49.0	34.84		
59.5	74.34	49.5	35.02		
60.0	75.39	50.0	35.56		

(Adapted from *Thin So Fast* by Dr Michael Eades [Warner Books, New York, 1989])

exercises that are relevant to your present muscular strength and endurance levels. There are two tests you need to carry out:

- The press-up test. Do as many continuous press-ups you can.
- The sit-up test. See how many curl-ups you can complete in a minute.

The press-up test
- Men – do full press-ups (see page 157)
- Women – do half press-ups (see page 155)

Carry out the exercise in the correct manner, as described in Chapter 14. Count each one. As soon as you are too tired to perform another repetition, note your score. Then find out your rating from the table below and record it.

Women					
Age	Poor	Fair	Average	Good	Excellent
10–20	<5	5–15	16–32	33–47	48+
20–30	<3	3–10	11–23	24–38	39+
30–40	<2	2–6	7–18	19–33	34+
40–50	<1	1–4	5–13	14–28	79+
50+	<0	0–1	2–8	9–18	19+

Men					
Age	Poor	Fair	Average	Good	Excellent
10–20	<19	19–33	34–43	44–53	54+
20–30	<14	14–23	24–35	34–43	44+
30–40	<11	11–18	19–28	29–38	39+
40–50	<7	7–13	14–23	24–33	34+
50+	<4	4–8	9–18	19–28	29+

Now take your rating and see how many points you get for your rating in the chart below:

Poor	Fair	Average	Good	Excellent
0	2	3	4	6

Record that score. You'll need it later on.

The sit-up test
The test is to perform as many sit-ups as you can in 60 seconds, making sure your form is perfect throughout.

The exercise

Lie on your back, face up, with your stomach pulled in and back flattened. Your knees should be bent with your feet 30 to 60 cm (1 to 2 feet) from your backside. Place your hands either side of your head near your ears. Now curl your head and shoulders up off the floor and with your elbows touch your mid-thighs. Return to the start position ensuring your shoulders touch the floor each time. If you find your feet rise up, get a friend to hold your heels to stop this. Do not let them hold the top of your feet; this nullifies the difficulty of the exercise.

When you do the exercise do not pull yourself up with your arms. Allow your stomach to do the work.

Use the table below to find out your rating.

Women

Age	Poor	Fair	Average	Good	Excellent
10–20	<33	33–36	37–42	43–47	48+
20–30	<25	25–28	29–34	35–39	40+
30–40	<20	20–22	23–29	30–34	35+
40–50	<15	15–18	19–24	25–29	30+
50+	<13	13–16	17–19	20–24	25+

Men

Age	Poor	Fair	Average	Good	Excellent
10–20	<37	37–40	41–46	47–51	52+
20–30	<29	29–32	33–38	39–43	44+
30–40	<24	24–27	28–33	34–38	39+
40–50	<19	19–22	23–28	29–33	34+
50+	<14	14–17	18–23	24–28	29+

Record your score in points.

Poor	Fair	Average	Good	Excellent
0	2	3	4	6

Now take the two scores – your points from the press-up test and the sit-up test – and add them together. The result will indicate which strength-training programme you should use as a starting-point. (These programmes are outlined in Chapter 14.)

- If your score is between 0 and 6 choose Programme 1 exercises from the strength-training menu.
- If your score is between 7 and 12, choose Programme 2 exercises from the strength-training menu.

Flexibility test

The flexibility test is designed to measure flexibility in your hamstring muscles (the ones in the back of your thigh) and lower back. Good flexibility is important in relation to co-ordination and prevention of injury. A full range of motion around a joint will guard against torn or stretched ligaments and tendons.

The test

Make sure your body is warmed up and stretched before taking this test. Put a tape-measure on the floor and stick some tape across it at the 38-cm (15-inch) point. Further unroll it to about 1 metre (39½ inches) and stick tape across it again. Sit with your heels at the 38-cm point, facing in the direction of the 1-metre point. Ensure your feet are about 25 cm (10 inches) apart and your toes are pointing towards the ceiling. Curl your trunk forward with your fingers outstretched. Reach as far forward as you can. Do not bounce into the stretch, but maintain control at all times. Hold the stretch at the furthest point for 3 seconds and note which measurement on the tape you reach with your fingertips. Repeat the process once more. Work out the average of the two results.

Now, using the table below, record your score.

Women	under 35		36–45		46+	
	cm	inches	cm	inches	cm	inches
Excellent	58.5	23	58.5	23	56	22
Good	53.5	21	53.5	21	48	19
Average	45.5	18	43	17	38	15
Fair	35.5	14	30.5	12	28	11
Poor	28	11	25.5	10	23	9
Men	cm	inches	cm	inches	cm	inches
Excellent	53.5	21	56	22	51	20
Good	48	19	48	19	43	17
Average	38	15	35	14	33	13
Fair	25.5	10	28	11	23	9
Poor	17.5	7	12.5	5	12.5	5

Summary

By now you are in a position to choose the appropriate aerobic exercise and strength-training programme to start with. You know various body statistics about yourself and you know how good or bad your flexibility is.

It is a good idea to store all this information for future use. A chart is provided below. Redo the tests every 6 weeks. This is a long enough time for significant changes to have happened, but not so long that you forget why you began exercising in the first place.

Name... Age........ Date ....

Body measurements

chest/bust (over nipple line)   .... inches

biceps (relaxed state; widest point)
   right   .... inches
   left   .... inches

waist (over navel)   .... inches

hips (at widest point)   .... inches

top of thigh
   right   .... inches
   left   .... inches

calf (at widest point)
   right   .... inches
   left   .... inches

resting pulse (BPM)   ....

body-fat percentage   ....

total body weight   ....

body-fat weight   ....

lean muscle mass weight   ....

aerobic step test		sit-up test	
score	....	score	....
rating	....	rating	....
press-up test		flexibility test	
score	....	score	....
rating	....	rating	....

Sources of energy

When you start exercising regularly, it's important to know something about your body's needs in terms of energy. Your body has two main reservoirs of energy which are used under normal conditions. The first source is fat, which is by far the larger in terms of size.

A man weighing 81.5 kilos (180 pounds), with a body-fat percentage of 20, has about 16.5 kilos (36 pounds) of stored fat. Of that, all but about 1.5 kilos (3 pounds) is available to use as energy, leaving him with 15 kilos (33 pounds) for that purpose. Half a kilo (1 pound) of fat contains approximately 3500 calories, which means that the entire amount of energy available to him is 115,000 calories (33 x 3500). That's an amazing reservoir.

The other main source of energy is digested food. Your body can store between 1500 and 2000 calories of energy in its system, ready to be used when it's needed. By topping up, you can keep this source full to the brim, but the total usable amount will remain the same.

Your body has to be able to perform different functions at different levels of exertion. On one level, your body needs to carry out activities at a low rate of exertion for long periods of time. This is called living. This level covers the whole spectrum of activity, from watching television right up to jogging, skipping and other forms of cardiovascular exercise.

The other side of the equation is when you want your body to perform intensive explosive types of activity for short periods of time, like lifting heavy objects, or running very fast.

We're going back to our caveman to give you examples of all this.

When he sets off from his cave at a fast walking pace or a slow jog, the caveman is working in or below the aerobic zone. At this point he is fuelling his system with a combination of oxygen and proportional levels of fat and digested food energy. If he used only his food source, he would run out of his 2000 stored calories relatively quickly. But the body doesn't like doing this, so it supplies a cocktail of fat and food fuel, with the accent heavily on the fat part.

Once he finds a fierce animal, he closes in for the kill. His body needs to release large amounts of energy very quickly for this.

Because energy from fat is not as quickly released as energy from food fuel, his body switches to using mostly this type of fuel. This is called anaerobic fuelling, which means fuelling without air. This is extremely effective for periods of about 90 to 120 seconds. After that he needs to return to an aerobic level or stop.

This system evolved to support the 'fight or flight' level of activity of our ancestors' more dangerous existence, where it was essential for survival. Now we use it only occasionally, to run for the bus perhaps. But we still have the same systems.

The line between aerobic and anaerobic exercise is not as clearly defined as you might think. Quite a lot of activities are a combination of the two. This is especially true of sports such as tennis and squash, where the level of activity is likely to fluctuate quickly and often. With these games, it's hard to pick the correct rate for maximizing fat loss, because the rate of exertion changes so frequently. To achieve the best results, therefore, we need to be careful to specify exercises where the level of activity remains reasonably constant.

Our training programme (see Chapter 14) is designed specifically to make a rapid improvement in cardiovascular efficiency, and increase muscle tone and strength.

In short, our conclusions are:

- When working aerobically or sub-aerobically our bodies draw on proportionately larger percentages of fat fuel.
- When we're in anaerobic mode, our body fuels the exertion with higher levels of food fuel.

Training zones and heart rate

You can quantify your aerobic and anaerobic 'zones' of activity (i.e. how hard you should be exercising) by measuring your heart rate. First you need to know what your maximum heart rate is. You can then work out the appropriate zone as a percentage of that figure.

The maximum heart rate

This is imaginatively referred to as Max HR. No amount of exercise will increase the heart rate above this level. In fact, further exercise may burst the heart, especially if you haven't been using it much at this level.

With Max HR it is important to work out the number of beats that work for you, and this will vary with age and fitness. A very fit person can be asked to run or cycle flat out for four or five minutes, and then their maximum heart rate can be measured. For someone who is not so fit, this procedure is dangerous.

Rather than do that, we are going to use an age-adjusted formula:

For men:	Subtract your age from 220.
	The result is your maximum heart rate.
	(For example, a 40-year-old man may have a Max HR of 180.)
For women:	Subtract your age from 226.
	The result is your maximum heart rate.
	(For example, a 40-year-old woman may have a Max HR of 186.)

Percentages of your maximum heart rate can be used to work out training zones aimed at achieving specific effects on the body. These might be:

- weight reduction
- cardiovascular fitness
- increased muscle mass.

We have combined several possible zones for the purpose of this book:

- **Zone 1** – exercise-introduction and weight-management zone. In this zone you exercise at 55 to 70 per cent of your Max HR.
- **Zone 2** – cardiovascular zone. Here your heart rate is 70 to 80 per cent of your Max HR.
- **Zone 3** – anaerobic zone. The first 90 seconds of muscle-intensive exercise, performed at 80 to 100 percent of your Max HR.

Beats per minute (BPM)

To find out the heartbeats per minute (BPM) for each zone that are appropriate for you, multiply your Max HR by the zone's upper and lower percentage. (See the example below.)

The following calculations are based on the example of a 40-year-old man with a Max HR of 180 (220 – 40 = 180 Max HR). Substitute your own Max HR to work out your personal BPM for each zone level.

- **Zone 1** (55–70 per cent of Max HR)
  180 x 55 per cent (.55) = 99 BPM to
  180 x 70 per cent (0.70) = 126 BPM

- **Zone 2** (70–85 per cent of Max HR)
  180 x 70 per cent (0.70) = 126 BPM to
  180 x 85 per cent (0.85) = 153 BPM

- **Zone 3** (85–100 per cent of Max HR)
  180 x 85 per cent (0.85) = 153 BPM to
  180 x 100 per cent (100) = 180 BPM

Zone 1: exercise-introduction and weight-reducing zone

The point about this zone is that, although the exercise rate is low and you are barely working aerobically, the number of calories you burn is low but the proportion of fat fuel (as opposed to food fuel) you burn is high. Remember the word 'proportion' because it is important. If the number of calories burnt is low, the proportion of fat burnt is also low.

If you go walking for 20 minutes, you don't burn that many calories and therefore you don't burn much fat. This zone relies on duration to be effective. Golf is a sport which doesn't rely on high-heart rate levels. If done enough, say three 18-hole sessions a week, it will burn more fat than three 20-minute sessions of fast aerobic exercise, like running, a week. However, the golf will take up six to eight hours and the other exercise 60 minutes, so in terms of time it is quite costly. (And you have to wear stupid jumpers as well.)

What is zone 1 good for?

This rate of exercise is good for people who are just starting out on a weight-loss programme, who haven't exercised for many years and might have poor eating habits and smoke and drink too much. The risk from muscular injury at this rate is low, and because it's not excessively hard, it isn't painful either.

It's also good for people who used to be fitter and need to get back into their exercise routine gradually. Lastly, it is good for people who are a bit older and don't want to use the higher-intensity rates to accomplish what they need. Remember, to increase your health dramatically you don't need to bust a gut.

How to do it

Because your heart rate is low in this zone, anything that is going to make your heart beat faster than this level will not be practical. These activities are suitable at this rate:

- walking and fast walking (on a treadmill or outside)
- swimming
- slow cycling
- golf
- mowing the lawn.

How long do I do it for?

Because of the low number of calories you burn per hour, you unfortunately have to go for duration. This means realistically two to four hours a week, but start on half that. This seems impossible for some people with busy schedules. Here are some suggestions to overcome this problem:

- Cycle to and from work.
- If you drive and cannot do otherwise, park a few kilometres away from the office and walk in.
- Set out early for appointments and walk to them.
- Use weekends for walks, swims or cycle rides.
- Use stairs instead of escalators and lifts on the underground or in office blocks.
- Use your lunch break to go out and exercise.
- Don't use your car for short journeys unless unavoidable.

If you can do some or all of these things, it's amazing how quickly the hours mount up. Keep a careful record and try to exercise over 20 minutes each time, and preferably for about 40 minutes. If you fall short regularly, take steps to make up the time in scheduled exercise sessions.

Zone 2: the cardiovascular or aerobic zone

Working within the aerobic zone maximizes benefits to your cardiovascular system. Your perceived rate of exertion will be greater than the last zone. It will feel quite hard, but you should still retain control. This is not the rate to start at if you haven't been exercising for a while.

In terms of fat-burning, proportionally you are now burning more food fuel than fat fuel. However, the number of calories you are burning is higher, so don't think you aren't burning the fat. Indeed, when Richard trains people who are pretty fit, this is the rate he uses to burn fat, although he keeps his clients at the lower end of this zone. If you look at this equation you will see why:

Burning fat – low or high intensity

EXERCISE INTENSITY	Less intense	More intense
	30 minutes of exercise at 50% of max HR	30 minutes exercise at 75% of max HR
Result	More fat burned, 50% from fat per single calorie	Less fat burned, 40% from fat per single calorie
Total cals used	225	315
Total fat cals used	113	126

The increased intensity of Zone 2 as opposed to Zone 1 burns more body fat. But if you're a beginner, work in Zone 1 until you're fit enough to work in Zone 2. This will avoid you getting injured or discouraged.

The other benefit of the aerobic zone is that it elevates your metabolism significantly for up to six hours after exercising. The body becomes like a train that runs fast for a while and then switches off its engine. Afterwards, it will continue to go for some time. It also produces aerobic enzymes that are designed to help metabolize fat.

The body adapts, as we have said before, to help you to be more efficient, so if you regularly remind it that it has to do this type of exertion, it will respond in this way.

Aerobic enzymes are produced in the first zone as well as the second, but to a lesser degree. Therefore it is advisable regularly to exercise at a sub-aerobic (Zone 1) or aerobic exercise (Zone 2) level.

What is Zone 2 for?

This type of exercise is good for people going on from Zone 1 who want to benefit from the cardiovascular aspect as well. You must work up to it gradually, and extend the duration of the exercise sessions gradually too.

How to do it

All these are good Zone 2 activities:

- jogging
- fast walking
- cycling quite fast
- swimming quite fast
- rollerblading
- canoeing (fine if you can organize it)
- aerobics (but difficult to control your heart rate here)
- step machines, or steps outside or bench-stepping (very boring, though)
- cross-country skiing machine.

How long do I do it for?

Work first in Zone 1 and then have a five-minute foray into Zone 2. Then, as long as you feel OK, incrementally extend the duration over a period of, say, one month. You should eventually be doing three to four weekly sessions of 30 to 45 minutes at a time, totalling an hour and a half to 2 hours a week. This will, in conjunction with eating properly, give you a solid base of fitness and low body-fat level.

Zone 3: anaerobic zone

This zone is unusual in that it uses both ends of the spectrum. During the first second or two of exercise, the muscles principally draw on energy stores located within themselves. These sources are anaerobic, meaning no air, since they make no use of oxygen in producing energy.

First the muscles tap a substance called ATP (adenosine triphosphate), the only fuel that can directly fuel a muscle. The stored supply is minuscule and burns out in a second. Another phosphate compound in the muscle, creating phosphate, is used to synthesize a fresh supply of ATP. This lasts for about another ten seconds when the exertion rate is high.

After that the muscle begins to use a third energy source, glycogen or food fuel, converted from the glucose in starches and sugars. This is then converted into ATP during a process called anaerobic glycolysis which supplies the quick energy. But the process stops after about 90 seconds because of a by-product called lactic acid that accumulates in muscles and causes them to fatigue.

You can see why weight-training, which lasts for only short periods, and a person who gradually increases his running speed till he is sprinting are both in the anaerobic zone. The fuel used comes almost entirely from food and not from the body's fat reserves. People who work in this zone tend to build muscle mass with it, because it is a muscle-intensive zone. Essentially they are working the muscles to overload. When this happens, the body registers that it needs to be stronger to deal with the stimuli it is receiving. Look at sprinters' legs or the muscles of a body-builder and you will see the extreme results of this principle.

What is it good for?

The more muscle you have, the more calories you burn per hour within your standard metabolic rate. Allied to correct eating, this will reduce your proportion of body-fat. Additionally, when you build muscle you manufacture something called human growth hormone. This hormone is central to the reconstruction of muscle fibre into a bigger and better form after muscle-intensive exercise.

The energy that is used to fund this process comes from body fat. So by training anaerobically, especially in an activity that specifically targets muscles by overloading them, like weight-training, you can help reduce your body-fat levels.

Richard doesn't usually get clients to train in the high heart rate anaerobic zone unless it's for a specific need – for instance, if they have to run fast in a film. Working at this level can lead to muscular injuries. Muscle tone and size can be more safely gained through weight-training, which is something we will be doing. (When we say 'we' we mean you, of course.)

How to do it

The quickest way to gain either muscle tone or mass is to work with weights. This does not mean lifting large iron blocks around.

We will be using light weights to reduce injury risk and go for high repetitions.

How long do I do it for?

The idea of building large amounts of muscle mass is outside the parameters of this book, as it is a specialized field separate from weight loss and health maintenance. To produce good muscle tone over a period of six months will take approximately three to four sessions a week of about 45 to 60 minutes each time. Intensity at the beginning however will have to be worked up to slowly, to minimize the risk of injury.

Choosing your aerobic exercise

Choosing an exercise to burn fat or improve cardiovascular efficiency is not as simple a job as it at first appears. Books that show you how many calories are used up by different exercises are not giving you the whole story. Burning calories is a factor in exercise, but it isn't by any means the only one. Consider the following suggestions (listed in ascending order of priority):

1. Match the exercise to the heart rate you're trying to achieve. If you want to exercise in Zone 1, for example, running is not appropriate because it is too hard and you will find it almost impossible to stay within the 55 to 70 per cent range. That is why walking and slow cycling are more suitable. Similarly, working at the top end of Zone 2 (70 to 85 per cent) is difficult to achieve with a walk, although not impossible.
2. Pick an exercise, or exercises, that are convenient for you to do. Swimming is fine if you don't have to drive for an hour to get to a pool. Make your exercise 'user-friendly', so your training sessions do not have all the logistic requirements of launching the second front.
3. Pick an exercise that ties in with your physical condition. If you have a history of lower-back pain, stay away from exercises that could jar it, like running or aerobics. Instead, go swimming, cycling, walking or use a step machine.
4. Most importantly, pick a form of exercise you enjoy. That way it will be a pleasure and you will be more inclined to do it.

Remember, there is no law which says you should train with only one type of exercise. By switching from one to another you actually give your body a better work-out and enhance the training effect. As the saying goes, variety is the spice of life.

Sports training

Sports are great: they get you out of the house, they relieve stress, they are fun, they're social and they offer health benefits. But, in terms of producing specific weight-loss results, building muscle tone and being controllable, they are not necessarily that effective.

Your heart rate, depending on the sport, will flip in and out of zones and won't always produce the results you want. Sport is an important aspect of being healthy but should be treated separately from your fitness programme. Once you have achieved your goals with us, you may decide to substitute sports sessions for our training sessions, but initially you should follow the programme outlined in this book.

How to measure your heart rate

With Zone 1 and 2 exercise, you need to be able to measure your heart rate in order to maximize benefits from the programme. You can use one of these two methods:

1. Take your heart rate while exercising from your pulse, at your wrist or at your neck. Count for six seconds and then multiply by ten to give you your beats per minute (BPM). You will need to stop to do this, which is not ideal. Alternatively, you can use a heart-rate monitor, which is easier since you don't need to stop at all. Heart-rate monitors are expensive, though, costing £60 to £150. (You should buy one, however, because you need it.)

   Most heart-rate monitors can be pre-set to the zone you want to exercise in. They will warn you by an audible beep that you are outside your required zone, which allows you to speed up or slow down if necessary. This is ideal for our purposes.
2. The second way relies on perceiving your rate of exertion. With this approach, you rate on a numerical scale how strenuous you feel your exercise is. The chart below shows the likely correlation between what you feel and the zone percentages.

Method 2

Perceived level of exertion	Percentage of max hr	Effects on you
1 Very easy	55%	Very comfortable
2 Quite easy	60%	Can hold a normal conversation without gasping
3 Moderate	70%	Can speak short sentences without gasping
4 Quite hard	75%	Short sentences make you gasp a little
5 Hard	80%	Speaking more than a few words is difficult
6 7 8 9 Very hard	85%	You don't want to talk
10 Extremely hard	85–100%	Extremely unpleasant

Remember, as you get fitter you will move faster, without necessarily raising your heart rate. Your rating of perceived exertion is therefore accurate, to a certain extent, because you are gauging your exercise by exertion, rather than the speed you move. The term 'Listen to your body' is relevant here.

Aims of the programme

The programme outlined in this book is designed to accomplish the following:

- reduce body fat percentages
- increase cardiovascular efficiency
- increase muscle tone and some muscle mass
- increase flexibility.

These are specific aims which will cover what most people want from exercise. Anything further would require adjusting the programme and an assessment should be made when it is completed. Our programme is relevant in terms of other fitness pursuits. If you want to run a marathon, for example, the programme will create a useful fitness platform to start from. It is also a good starter programme for those who want to increase their muscle mass to a significant degree.

14
Getting Down To It

We've reached a point where you have to put up or shut up. We've laid out a few pointers to help you make the decision to start exercising. Make sure you read this whole chapter before you start the training programme. It could – and probably will – make the difference between success and failure for you.

Rules for training

Always follow the following rules about training:

- Assess your fitness.
- Wear appropriate training clothes and footwear.
- Start slowly.
- Warm up before stretching.
- Cool down after exercise.
- Stretch before exercise (and sometimes even during).
- Train safely.

Assess your fitness

Before you embark on a fitness programme, you need to assess your starting-point, so that you begin training at a level which is safe, enjoyable and reasonable. If you don't get this equation right you can quickly become dispirited and stop.

On pages 116–125 you will find a simple fitness assessment which you must do so that the different levels of training in the next chapter will make sense. Also included is a list of body measurements you should record and store so comparisons can be made with the new you further down the road.

Wear appropriate training clothes and footwear

By far the most important item you will buy is your trainers. They must be appropriate to the exercises you are doing. Buy the best ones you can afford. There are plenty of big stores that specialize in this sort of thing and the assistants are trained to be helpful. Explain what exercises you will be doing and choose your trainers on the basis of their advice.

Make sure that your clothes are loose enough not to restrict movement. Wear layers of clothing that you can put on or take off according to the weather and the heat you generate when training.

Start slowly

A sudden burst of activity after a few years of sedentary living could lead to injury. Minor muscular aches and twinges are normal but severe muscular discomfort or excessive cardiovascular strain are not. So work into the exercise programme gradually. If you're starting your programme by using Zone 1, halve the recommended training time of two to four hours a week to one to two hours a week to begin with, and then build up. Once you're happy at the minimum number of hours, gradually increase it to the maximum number.

Look at the ranges in the zones. Zone 1 is 55 to 70 per cent and Zone 2, 70 to 85 per cent. Again, start working at the bottom end of the zone and gradually increase the rate to the higher end.

With your weight-training programme there are minimum repetition and maximum repetition numbers. Start at the lower end and work up. Once you're used to the weight at the top number of repetitions, increase the weight and drop the number of repetitions to a manageable number. Then go up again or even enter Zone 2 where the exercises are harder. But, again, start at the bottom.

Warm up before stretching

Before exercising or stretching you must warm up your body. By this we mean exercising quite lightly, using your large muscle groups to about 50 to 60 per cent of your maximum heart rate. Basically, you should work up a slight sweat. You can do this by cycling, walking, jogging, marching on the spot or light aerobic movement exercises. Warming up prepares your heart, joints and muscles for what is to come. It should take about five minutes.

Cool down after exercise

Whichever type of exercise you are doing, spend five minutes at the end cooling down and relaxing. Then do your stretches.

Stretch before exercise (and sometimes even during)

Flexibility is a measure of fitness, just as strength and cardiovascular efficiency and endurance are. It must be included in your training programme. Flexibility promotes good posture, minimizes risk from muscular injury, increases the range of motion of your limbs and lengthens the muscle, giving it a well-proportioned appearance.

Flexibility is increased by stretching muscles. It should be done on a daily basis, even on days when you are resting from other parts of the programme. It should be done before and after you train, whether you are working aerobically or with weights. With weights you should stretch after each exercise to allow your blood to carry away any lactic acid build-up which can inhibit your performance.

Apart from stretching in conjunction with your training programme you should try to do some simple stretches first thing in the morning and last thing at night. By doing this you start and end each day on a positive note, which is good for morale. Think of it this way: if you spend fifteen minutes stretching on waking you are less likely to pig out on the wrong sort of breakfast.

A detailed stretching routine is illustrated on the following pages. Ensure you get to grips with it. It is important.

Stretching

The following stretching routine is a multi-purpose one. It is used for aerobic Zones 1 and 2 and weight-training.

For Zones 1 and 2, after your warm-up complete the routine. Having finished exercising, stretch again before you shower. The only difference with a weight routine is that you should also stretch individual muscles after each set, because you can become over-tight. Otherwise, by the time you get to your stretch at the end, it can take much longer. Use some or all of the stretches for your morning and evening stretch as well.

Stretching routine

hip and back stretch
hamstring stretch
groin stretch
front of thigh stretch
calf stretch
lower back and abdominal
   stretch (cat stretch)

lower back stretch
side stretch
chest and biceps stretch
triceps stretch
shoulder stretch
shoulder shrug
neck stretch

Hip and back stretch

Stretches: hips, outer thighs, lower back
and outer abdominals

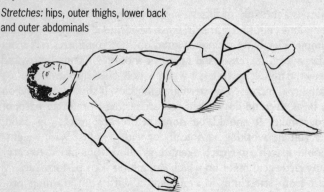

Lie on the floor with both legs bent and knees raised. Contract your stomach muscles and flatten your back, keeping your head down, your neck relaxed and your eyes above. Place your right thigh over your left and let the weight of the right thigh slowly carry the left thigh towards the ground. Ensure you keep both your shoulders and hips in contact with the ground. Pause for 20–30 seconds, breathing steadily. Slowly return to the upright position. Now put your left thigh over the right thigh and repeat.

Hamstring stretch

Stretches: back of thigh and part of calf muscle

Find a low wall or stable chair and stand square to it. Place one leg on it so that it comes about half-way up your calf. Placing both hands on the top of the raised leg, breathe out and slowly move the upper half of your body towards your thigh. Keep your back straight. Once you feel the stretch in the back of your thigh, use your hands to stay in that position. Stay in this position for 20–30 seconds, breathing regularly. If you feel you can push further into the stretch, breathe out as you do it. Do not over-stretch. Pull out of the stretch by straightening your arms. Change legs and repeat.

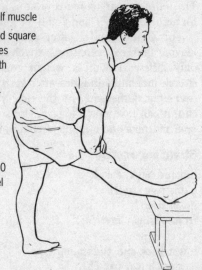

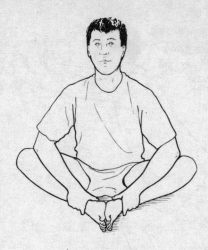

Groin stretch

Stretches: inside of thigh and lower back

Sit on the floor with your legs out in a V, then draw together the balls of your feet with your heels towards your groin. Then place your hands on your ankles and your elbows on your knees and carefully press down on knees until the inside thigh muscles are comfortably stretched, which will take about 20 to 30 seconds. Relax and breathe steadily. Slowly return to the starting position.

Front of thigh stretch

Stretches: front of thigh (quadriceps)

Stand with your feet shoulder width apart, and use your left arm to balance against a wall or chair. Transfer your weight to the left leg, bend the left knee slightly and tuck the buttocks under. Bring your right heel back and lift it up towards the buttocks, reaching for the ankle with your right hand. Use your right arm to bring the heel further up into the stretch. Hold for 20 to 30 seconds, then lower the right leg and repeat the process with the left.

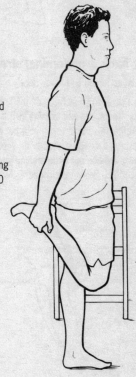

Calf stretch

Stretches: calves (gastrocnemius and soleus muscles)

Stand 90 cm to 1 metre (about 3 feet) away from a wall, with your body and toes facing it. Put your right foot forward with the knee bent to stretch the soleus muscle. Keep the left (rear) knee straight, to stretch gastrocnemius muscle. Place your hands flat against the wall about shoulder width apart, keeping your heels planted. Then slowly lean towards the wall by bending the elbows. Pause for 20–30 seconds in a comfortably stretched position. Relax and breathe regularly. Return to the starting position, change legs and repeat.

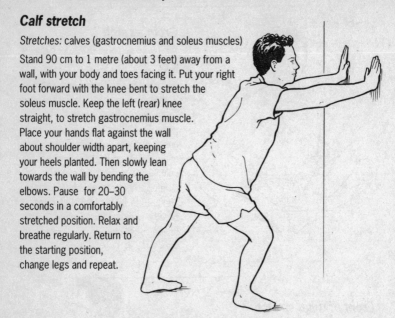

Lower back & abdominal stretch (cat stretch)

Stretches: abdomen and lower back

Take up a position on all fours on the floor, with your hands shoulder width apart. Hold your stomach in and breathe in. Tilt your head till your eyes are looking straight ahead. At the same times arch your back gently. Hold for 10 seconds. Once the back is comfortably arched, start to bring your head down till your chin is near the front of your chest. Breathe out while arching your back upwards (the reverse position). Hold for 10 seconds. Repeat the process three times.

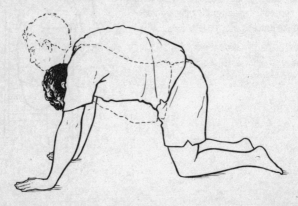

Lower back stretch

Stretches: lower back

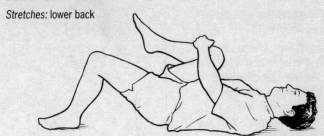

Lie on the ground with both knees bent. Push the small of the back flat to the ground. Lift the right leg, with the knee still bent, towards your chest. Form a circle with your arms around the knee and pull it gently towards you. Hold the stretched position, breathing naturally, for 20 to 30 seconds. Then gently release. Repeat with your other leg.

Side stretch

Stretches: outer back (latissimus dorsae) and outer abdominals

Stand with your feet shoulder width apart. Put your arms above your head with your arms as close to your ears as possible. Looking straight ahead and breathing out slowly, bend your upper body over to one side till you feel the stretch. Hold for 15 to 20 seconds, breathing normally. Slowly bring your body up to the vertical and repeat the process on the other side.

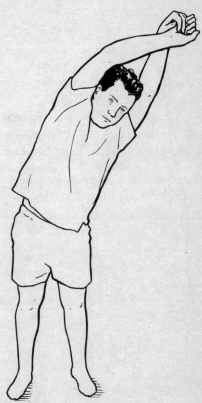

Chest and biceps stretch

Stretches: chest muscles and biceps
(front of upper arm)

Find an upright post (e.g. a door-frame)
that is at least shoulder height. Place
your right hand flat against the left side
of the post so that your palm faces to
the right. Now move your body in a
clockwise direction, staying in the same
spot, so that you stretch the biceps
and chest muscles. Once you reach a
comfortable but stretched position hold
it for 20 to 30 seconds. Reverse the
procedure and then stretch the other
side.

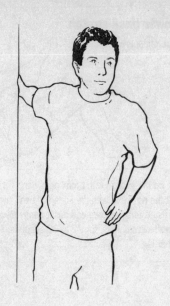

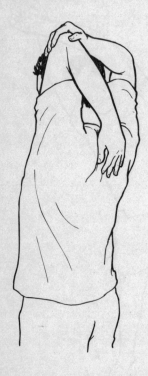

Triceps stretch

Stretches: triceps (back of upper arm) and
upper back

Stand with your feet slightly wider than your
shoulders. Keep your knees slightly bent.
Contract the abdominals and flatten your back.
Looking straight ahead, place your left forearm
behind your head, with your upper arm against
your ear. Lightly grasp your left elbow with your
right hand, then walk your hand down your spine
to a comfortable stretched position. Pause, relax
and breathe evenly for 20 seconds. Slowly return
to the starting position and repeat with other
side.

Shoulder stretch

Stretches: shoulder muscles (deltoids)

Stand with your feet shoulder width apart and your knees slightly bent. Contract your abdominals and flatten your back. Place your right arm across your chest. Now put your left hand against your right elbow and push gently towards your chest till you get a comfortable stretch. Breathe naturally and hold for 20 seconds. Slowly release from the stretch and repeat the process with the other arm.

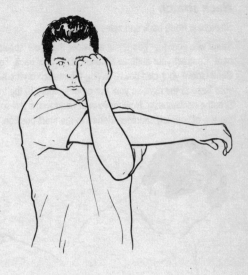

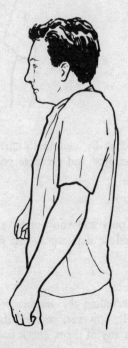

Shoulder shrugs

Stretches: middle of upper back (trapezius) and neck

Stand with your feet apart, slightly wider than your shoulders, and knees slightly bent. Contract your abdominals and flatten your back. Focus your eyes straight ahead. Gently raise both shoulders towards your ears, pause and breathe regularly. Move your shoulders down, not to the fully stretched position, then pause, relax and breathe continuously. Repeat ten times. Then repeat ten times with the right shoulder only, moving it counter-clockwise. Repeat ten times with the left shoulder only, moving it counter-clockwise.

Neck stretch

Stretches: front, back and sides of neck

Stand with your feet apart, slightly wider than your shoulders, and your knees slightly bent. Contract your abdominals and flatten your back. Focus your eyes straight ahead. Gently move your chin down, feeling the stretch on the back of the neck. Now move your head to the right so your ear comes closer to the top of your right shoulder. Breathe continuously. Now move your head to the left so your left ear comes closer to the top of your left shoulder. Return to the start position. Repeat five times.

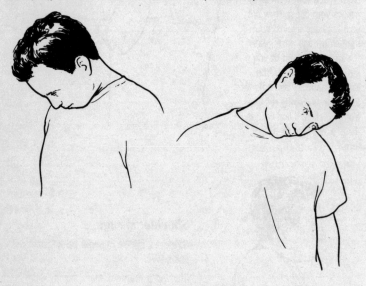

All the above are basic but effective stretches. By continually carrying them out you will increase your flexibility and decrease your chances of pulling muscles. So do them!

Feeling ill

If you don't feel well, don't train. Not only will you not have a good session, but certain exercises would be dangerous. Just get better and pick the programme up later.

Train safely

All the exercises shown in this book, including the aerobic programmes, are safe and uncontroversial. If, however, you feel that something is not right while carrying out any of them, check back to the book and see if you are doing it right. If you are and it still doesn't feel right, do an alternative exercise.

Guidelines for training

You will benefit from considering the following points. They are not rules, but suggestions to help you succeed with your fitness training.

* Make a declaration of intent.
* Get a training partner.
* Think positive.
* Set aside time and space to train.
* Don't panic if you miss training.
* Enjoy yourself.

Make a declaration of intent

Write down on a piece of paper a declaration of intent. It should just say something like 'I am going to enter into the training and eating regime with 100 per cent determination and do the very best I can.' That's all. (You can store it with your fitness assessment results.) By doing this – and meaning it – you are declaring to yourself how much it means to you. My experience is that people who try to avoid signing a declaration like this are generally the ones who fail, because their heart isn't in it. Richard made me sign one, and you feel really committed once you have written it down. This is the moment you start to go for it.

Get a training partner

Initially at least, training with someone else makes a project like this (for 'project' read 'the rest of your life') much easier. When one weakens, the other is strong and vice versa. A partner can be anyone: your husband or wife, a business partner, your oldest child – anyone who is part of your life and wants to get to grips with his or her health in a constructive way.

Think positive

We all meet people who are on some kind of fitness or nutrition regime and spend their whole time being miserable about it. You know by listening to them for five minutes that they view everything they do as a pain. They are fighting the very thing they're trying to achieve. But you, you're going to try to begin each day by reaffirming your intent to succeed. This isn't bullshit, it works. Point out to yourself that you feel better and you look better and remind yourself of all the other positive aspects of the deal. Learn to be at one with this feeling. It's a friend.

Set aside time and space to train

If exercise becomes the last priority in your life, you'll never do it. Like any other appointment, it needs to be scheduled. Be firm with yourself. Richard has trained hundreds of businessmen and has yet to meet one who said their business suffered as a result of training. Generally, the opposite happens.

If you're exercising at home, try to organize the area where you train so it's user-friendly. Clear a space that is sufficient for your purpose. Move some of the clutter or toys out of the way. Put down a towel or mat if the area is not carpeted. Once you start training your entire focus should be on it and a clear space helps.

Don't panic if you miss training

We've kept on about how you must keep going and stick to the programme. Sometimes, however, events in your life make this virtually impossible. When this happens, prioritize your life and see how things stack up against your training. If exercise has to lose out, so be it. Do as much as you can, but don't kill yourself. Get back to it as soon as possible. But try to be good about your food even when you're not exercising. That way you can maintain some balance.

Enjoy yourself

Above all, for God's sake, *enjoy it*. Enjoy having renewed energy, a better look, more self-respect and all the other stuff. It is not a prison sentence.

Progress

Finally, a word about progress. Progress in training is odd: the nearer you get to your goal the slower the process becomes. At the start of the season, an Olympic sprinter might knock off a second over 200 metres and then spend the rest of the season trying to knock a tenth of a second off that time. Don't be worried about progress; it will happen naturally in its own time.

15
Training Templates

Having done your assessment test and taken your body measurements, you are now in a position to start training. In order to use the templates, you must know whether you are on:

- aerobic training Zone 1 or Zone 2
- strength-training Programme 1 or Programme 2.

Aerobic training

The flowing progressive training schedule shows you how you can progress from Day 1 right up to the six-month point, where you go into maintenance mode for the rest of your life!

Choose your aerobic exercise from the exercise menu depending on whether you tested Zone 1 or Zone 2.

Week	times per week	minutes	% max hr	rpe*
Conditioning Base				
1	2–3	5–15	55–70%	2–4
2	2–3	5–15	55–70%	2–4
3	2–3	10–17	55–70%	2–4
4	2–3	10–17	55–70%	2–4
5	3	15–20	60–75%	2–4
6	3–4	15–20	60–75%	2–4
Improvement Stage				
7–9	3–4	20–25	60–75%	3–4
10–13	3–4	21–25	70–75%	4–5
14–16	3–4	26–30	70–75%	4–5
17–19	3–5	26–30	75–80%	4–5
20–23	3–5	31–35	75–80%	4–6
24–27	3–6	31–35	75–80%	4–6
Maintenance				
After 4–6 months	3–6	30–60	60–85	4–7

*rate of perceived exertion

Aerobic training rules

- Warm up and stretch before you exercise.
- Stretch and cool down after exercising.
- Train within your range (Zone 1: 55 to 70 per cent Max HR; Zone 2: 70 to 85 per cent Max HR).
- Remember, we live in the real world — obvious but true! If you have to rearrange your exercise days, just do it. But try to keep the spacings and timings the same if possible.
- Use walking and cycling (e.g. to and from work) as fillers to make up your exercise times.

Aerobic exercise menu

The following exercises are the main ones available without too much organization. Remember, on page 134 we gave you criteria for choosing.

Exercise	Advantages	Disadvantages	Zone 1/2	K CAL per hour
Walking/ race walking	• Good for beginners • Low injury rate – low impact • Conditions lower body but with weights and arm swinging good for upper body too. • Easy to organize • Can be done anywhere *Equipment* Good walking shoes	• Heart rate not easily elevated so progress can be slow • Calorific burn small so body fat reduction needs long periods of exercise	1	2 mph = 160 cals 4 mph = 360 cals 6 mph = 600 cals
Jogging or running	• Very efficient body conditioner and fat burner • Less time needed for results • Can be done anywhere • Beginners can combine walking and jogging to allow for poor stamina *Equipment* Best running shoes you can afford	• Impact on joints quite high so injury potential (see progressive training chart to minimize this or try soft surface running)	2	5 mph = 600 cals 6 mph = 700 cals 7 mph = 860 cals 9.5 mph = 1100 cals
Cycling	• Conditions upper and lower body • Low impact on joints • Can be incorporated into everyday life • Suitable for beginners or advanced *Equipment* A bike	• Can be dangerous • Can aggravate lower back problems (try recumbent indoor bikes) • Equipment can be expensive	1 or 2	Light 440 cals Moderate 550 cals Hard 750 cals V. hard 1000 cals

Exercise	Advantages	Disadvantages	Zone 1/2	K CAL per hour
Swimming	• Excellent whole-body conditioner • Very low injury rate • Suitable for joint/back problems *Equipment* Water, swimming trunks, goggles	• Requires access to water • Difficult to achieve sufficient heart rate if poor swimmer • Possibility of ear infection • Can be solitary	1 or 2	25 metres = 330 cals 40 metres = 480 cals 50 metres = 690 cals
Aerobics	• Good group type exercise • Much variety • Overall body conditioner • High/low impact types *Equipment* Good cross trainer shoes	• Doesn't suit everyone • Timing of classes cuts down flexibility • Difficult to maintain specific heart rate • Can be repetitive	2	Light 240 cals Moderate 400 cals Vigorous 600–1000 cals
Rowing	• Superb exercise for whole body • High calorific expenditure • Good at strengthening back *Equipment* Rowing machine or scull	• Access to equipment can be difficult • Equipment expensive • Can aggravate back problems	1 or 2	Light 400 cals Vigorous 840 cals
Aerobic circuit training *(star jumps, shadow boxing, marching on spot, jogging on spot, stepping, skipping)*	• Equipment needs minimal • Can be done anywhere • Highly aerobic • High calorific output if rest periods minimized • Suitable for hotel rooms *Equipment* Good stable running shoes, skipping rope, step or stairs	• Need to arrange easier exercises after hard ones so you don't go above your aerobic zone • Heart rate varies a lot	2	*Beginner's routine* 2 mins on, 30 seconds rest = 500 cals per hour *Advanced routine* 2 mins on, no rest = 1000 cals per hour

Practically anything is suitable as long as it makes you breathe harder so your pulse rate rises for long enough to an aerobic level. Dancing, gardening or walking the dog are all forms of exercise, too.

Strength-training

These templates need to be fitted in alongside your aerobic training sessions. There are different work-out routines for Programmes 1 and 2, and details of these are given after the templates.

Strength-training work-out routines

	Mon	Tues	Wed	Thurs	Fri	Sat	Sun
Programme 1	1	rest	2	rest	1	rest	2
Programme 2	1	rest	2	rest	3	rest	rest

Work-out routines

As the above table shows, you will perform different strength-training work-out routines on different days. The muscles you train in each work-out are listed below. Use the strength-training exercise menu on pages 153–154 to choose exercises appropriate to these muscles or muscle groups.

Programme 1

Work-out 1	*Work-out 2*
chest	front thigh and buttocks
front thigh and buttocks	outer obliques
shoulders	biceps
lower back	upper back
biceps	buttocks and rear of thigh
calves	obliques
triceps	shoulders
upper abdominals	chest
inner thigh	outer thigh
lower abdominals	triceps
hips	

Programme 2

Work-out 1	*Work-out 2*	*Work-out 3*
chest	front thigh and	shoulders
chest	buttocks	shoulders
chest	biceps	hips
upper abdominals	biceps	buttocks/rear of thigh
lower abdominals	lower back	buttocks/rear of thigh
upper back	triceps	upper back
calves	triceps	triceps
inner thigh	oblique abdominals	upper abdominals
outer thigh	outer oblique abdominals	lower abdominals

Strength-training instructions

On a strength-training day:

1. Find out which work-out routine you are doing.
2. Look up the muscle groups exercised by that routine.
3. Choose an appropriate exercise for each muscle group from the strength-training menu below.
4. Do two or three sets of each exercise.
5. For each set of upper-body exercises, do 10 to 20 repetitions. For each lower-body set, do 15 to 25 repetitions.

Other points:

- Always warm up and stretch before you train.
- Use weights where appropriate. The correct weight is one that makes the muscle you are working tired about two-thirds of the way through the set. By the last set, you should feel quite 'pumped' in the area you have been working.
- If you cannot complete the minimum number of repetitions, either do as many as you can while maintaining the correct form (you will improve!), or, if you are using weights, select a lighter one.
- Rest for 30 to 45 seconds between sets.
- The programme should take 45 to 60 minutes to complete.
- Remember to stretch and cool down when you have finished.

Strength-training exercise menu

Muscle Group	Exercise	Programme	Page
chest	box press-up	1	155
	half press-up	1	155
	bench press	1 and 2	156
	incline flye	1 and 2	156
	full press-up	2	157
shoulders	upright press	1 and 2	157
	lateral raise	1 and 2	157
	upright row	1 and 2	158
triceps	triceps press	1 and 2	158
	standing triceps extensions	1 and 2	159
	triceps dips	2	159
	triceps press-up	2	160

Muscle Group	Exercise	Programme	Page
biceps	biceps curl	1 and 2	160
	alternating curl	1 and 2	160
	split biceps curl (21's)	2	161
upper back	lying arm raise	1 and 2	161
	single arm row	1 and 2	162
	bent-over row	2	162
lower back	hyperextension	1 and 2	163
	lying alternate hyperextension	1 and 2	163
	kneeling alternate leg and arm raises	2	164
hips	seated knee-up	1 and 2	164
	hip roll	1 and 2	165
front thigh and buttocks	squat with support	1	165
	lunge with support	1	166
	squat without support	2	166
	lunge without support	2	166
buttocks and rear of thigh	lying back leg raise	1 and 2	167
hamstrings	back leg push	1 and 2	167
inner thighs	lying leg raise	1 and 2	168
outer thighs	side leg raise	1 and 2	168
calves	calf raise	1	169
	single-leg calf raise	2	169
upper abdominals	crunch	1	169
	crunch with legs raised	1 and 2	170
lower abdominals	reverse crunch	1 and 2	170
	alternate leg crunches	1 and 2	171
oblique abdominals	side crunch	1 and 2	171
	crunch twist	2	172
outer obliques	standing sidebend with pole	1	172
	standing sidebend with weights	2	172

Instructions on how to do the above exercises are given on the following pages.

Chest exercises

Box press-up

Assume a position on all fours (with a pad under your knees if necessary), with your hands a shoulder width apart. Hold in your stomach and tilt your pelvis so your back is not arched. Bend your arms till your forehead touches the ground and then push up again. Repeat. Breathe out on the way down. Breathe in on the way up.

Difficulty level – Programme 1

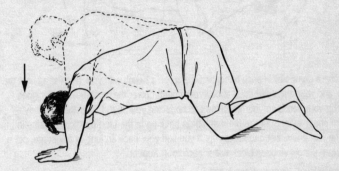

Half press-up

From the all-fours position, bring your hands forward so that your legs, back and head are in a straight line. Do not arch your back. Your hands should remain a shoulder width apart. Lower your body till your nose touches the floor, then raise it again. (Breathing, as for box press-up — see above.) Repeat.

Difficulty level – Programme 1

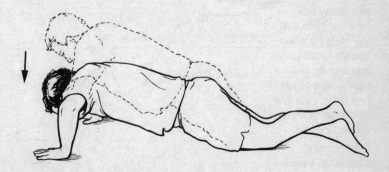

Bench press

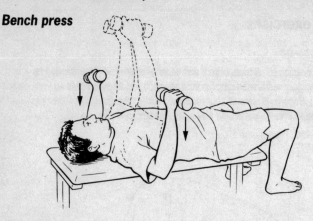

Holding a dumb-bell in each hand, lie face up on a bench with your feet flat against the floor and your arms extended above your chest. Lower the dumb-bells to the sides, turning your hands so your knuckles end up facing your feet. Lower them till they reach chest level. Squeeze the dumb-bells back up to the start position. Breathe in on the way down, out on the way up. If you find your back arching at any stage, put a 25-cm (10-inch) wooden block under each foot. Repeat.

Difficulty level – Programmes 1 and 2

Incline flye

Lie face up on a bench set at a 45-degree angle. Grasp a dumb-bell in each hand and hold with arms straight above your chest. Lower the dumb-bells slowly, flaring them to the sides until they are at chest level. Squeeze the dumb-bells back up to the first position. Again, if your back arches, raise your feet. Do not lock out your arms. Repeat.

Difficulty level – Programmes 1 and 2

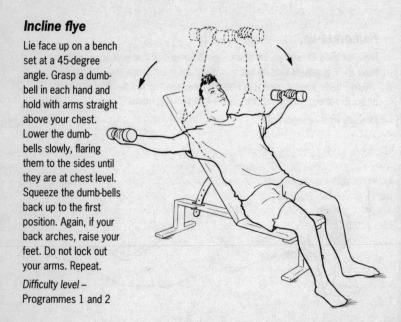

Full press-up

Lie face down on a mat. Place your hands directly under your shoulders and next to your chest. Keeping your body rigid and your legs, back and head in a straight line, straighten your arms until almost locked. Immediately lower yourself down till your chest brushes the floor. (Breathing, as for as box press-up – see page 155.) Repeat.

Difficulty level – Programme 2

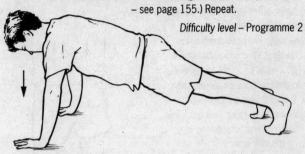

Shoulder exercises

Upright press

Sit on the end of a bench or a stable chair with a dumb-bell in each hand, held at shoulder level. Keeping your back straight and your eyes facing front, lift the weights until your arms are almost fully extended. Now lower the weights to the first position. Repeat. Breathe in on the way up and out on the way down.

Difficulty level – Programmes 1 and 2

Lateral raise

Stand upright, feet shoulder width apart, knees slightly bent, stomach pulled in and lower back flattened. Hold the dumb-bells on the front of your thighs, with your arms slightly bent and your hands facing inwards. Raise them till your hands are level with the top of your head. Make sure your elbows and hands stay roughly level throughout. Now lower your hands to the start position. Repeat. Breathe in on the way up and out on the way down.

Difficulty level – Programmes 1 and 2

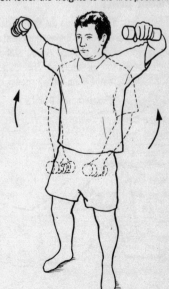

Upright row

Stand upright, with feet shoulder width apart, knees slightly bent, stomach held in and back flattened. Hold a dumb-bell in each hand, arms straight and palms facing your thighs. Lift both elbows simultaneously until both dumb-bells reach chin level. At chin height, elbows and hands should be at the same level. Lower to the first position slowly, then repeat. Do not heave on the weights when you are tired. Keep your back in a static position. Breathe in on the way up, out on the way down.

Difficulty level – programmes 1 and 2

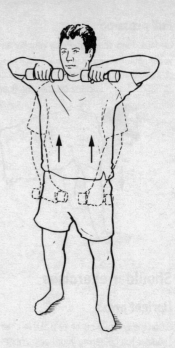

Triceps exercises

Triceps press

Lie face up on a bench or on the floor. Extend your arms with a dumb-bell in each hand so they are directly above your chest and your palms are facing your feet. Keeping your elbows and upper arms static, bend your elbows till the weights are lowered nearly to your forehead. Then straighten your arms again to return to the first position. Breathe in on the way down, out on the way up.

Difficulty level – Programmes 1 and 2

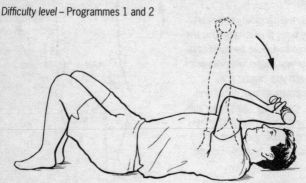

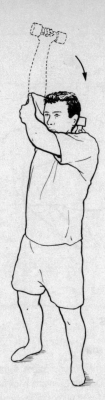

Standing triceps extensions

Stand with feet shoulder width apart, knees slightly bent, stomach pulled in and back flattened. Extend one arm straight up, holding the dumb-bell with the palm facing inwards. Brace your other hand against the underarm area of your extended arm. Now bend the extended arm so the dumb-bell moves down behind your head. Once there, straighten the arm, keeping the elbow locked in a static position braced with the stabilizing hand. Repeat. Breathe in on the way up and out on the way down.

Difficulty level – Programmes 1 and 2

Triceps dips

Sit on a sturdy bench or chair (make sure it won't move) or a low wall with your hands placed by your hips. Keeping your arms locked, extend your feet far enough so your bottom is just on the bench. Lower yourself till your upper arm is at 90 degrees to your lower arm. Raise yourself slowly till your arms are nearly locked, then repeat. Breathe in on the way up and out on the way down.

Difficulty level – Programme 2

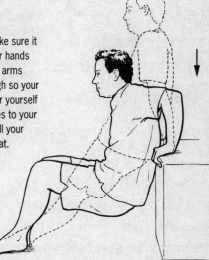

Triceps press-up

Assume the half press-up position
(see page 155) but with your hands
closer together, so they are about
7.5 cm (3 inches) apart. Lower and
raise as before, but keep your elbows
close to the sides of your body
throughout. Repeat. (Breathing: as
half press-up.)

Difficulty level – Programme 2

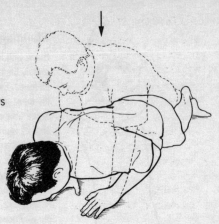

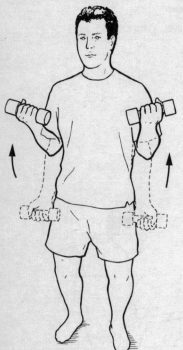

Biceps

Biceps curl

Stand upright with your knees slightly
bent, stomach pulled in and back flattened. Hold your dumb-bells by your side
with straight arms and your palms facing
forward. Curl both dumb-bells towards
your shoulders by flexing at the elbows.
Hold briefly, lower and then repeat.
Breathe in on the way up, out on the way
down.

Difficulty level – Programmes 1 and 2

Alternating curl

As for biceps curl (see above), but lift the dumb-bells alternately, not at the same time.

Difficulty level – Programmes 1 and 2

Split biceps curl (21's)

This exercise is a biceps curl in form, but to gain extra intensity it is split into three phases.

1. From the arms extended position, curl until you complete half of the movement, finishing with the weight in front of your waist. Do seven repetitions.
2. Without pausing, starting from the half-curl position, complete the remaining part of the curl, finishing with the weight opposite your shoulders. Do seven repetitions.
3. Without pausing, do seven repetitions of a compete biceps curl.

Difficulty level – Programme 2

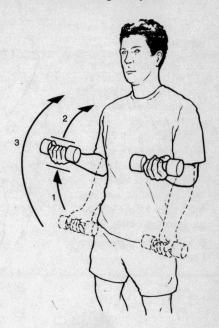

Upper back exercises

Lying arm raise

Lie face down. Bend both arms at a 90-degree angle and place them on the floor so the elbows are level with your shoulders. Keeping your head and hips in contact with the floor, slowly raise your bent arms off the floor, then lower them again. Repeat. Breathe in on the way up, out on the way down

Difficulty level – Programmes 1 and 2

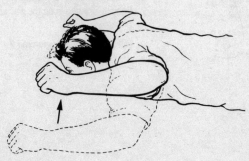

Single arm row

Stand beside a bench and place your left hand and knee on the bench with your right leg on the floor. Hold a dumb-bell in your right hand with your arm fully extended downward. Pull the weight upward to the side of your chest and hold for a count of 1. Slowly lower your arm to the starting position. Repeat. Then switch sides. Breathe in on the way up, out on the way down.

Difficulty level – Programmes 1 and 2

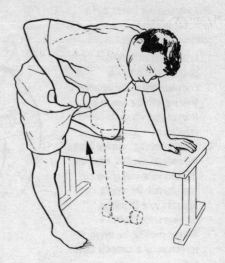

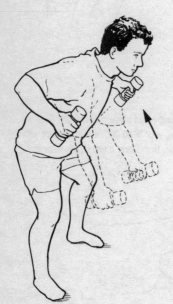

Bent-over row

Stand upright with a dumb-bell in each hand, held at arm's length. Slowly bend forward at the waist and lock your back, making sure you keep your knees slightly bent. Slowly pull the weights upwards to the sides of your chest. Slowly lower the weights until your arms straighten. Repeat. Breathe in on the way up and out on the way down.

Difficulty level – Programme 2

Lower back exercises

Hyperextension

Lie face down on a mat or on the floor with your hands on your backside, palm down. Slowly lift your head and upper back a few inches from the ground. Lower yourself slowly to the starting position. Breathe in on the way up, out on the way down.

Difficulty level – Programmes 1 and 2

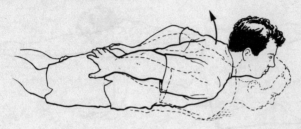

Lying alternate hyperextension

Lie face down on a mat or floor with both arms extended above your head and legs straight. Lift left arm and right leg a few inches from the ground and then slowly lower them. Now repeat, using your right arm and left leg. Your head will lift each time, but keep your eyes on the ground; do not arch your neck back. Breathe in on the way up and out on the way down.

Difficulty level – Programmes 1 and 2

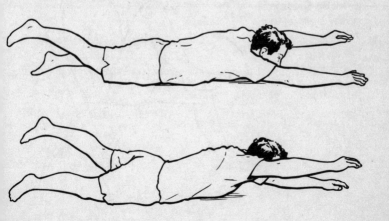

Kneeling alternate leg and arm raises

Get on all fours on a mat or the floor. Lift your right arm and extend it forward while extending your left leg back and up, parallel to the floor. Hold your leg and arm in the up position for a brief moment then lower to the starting position. Repeat with your left arm and right leg. Breathe in on the way up and out on the way down.

Difficulty level – Programme 2

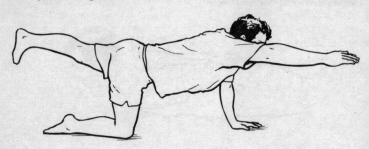

Hip exercises

Seated knee-ups

Sit on the edge of a chair or bench, holding both sides for stability. Lean slightly backwards and slowly lift your right knee towards your chest. Lower slowly and repeat with the left leg. Breathe in on the way up and out on the way down.

Difficulty level – Programmes 1 and 2

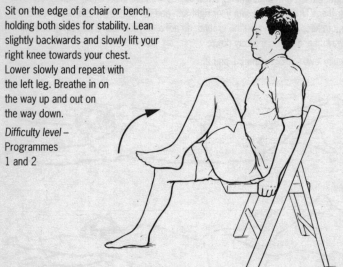

Hip roll

Stand upright at the end of a bench or chair (at least 30 cm/12 inches high) with your hands on your hips. Slowly lift the leg closest to the bench and swing it forward, then over the end around the bench. Repeat in the opposite direction by lifting your leg to the rear and swinging it over and around to the front of the bench. Switch sides and repeat. Breathe in on the way up and out on the way down.

Difficulty level –
Programmes
1 and 2

Front thigh (quadriceps) and buttocks exercises

Squat with support

Stand with feet shoulder width apart, knees slightly bent and your toes pointing slightly outward. Hold a pole (e.g. a broom-handle) about 60 cm (2 feet) in front of your feet, with both hands on the end of it. Slowly bend at your hips and knees to lower yourself until your thighs are parallel to the floor. Ensure your knees do not go any further forward than the tips of your toes. Hold the down position briefly and then rise to the start position. Use the pole to provide stability and a little leverage if necessary. Breathe out on the way down and in on the way up.

Difficulty level – Programme 1

Lunge with support

Stand upright with your feet shoulder width apart and your left hand by your side, pull in your stomach and flatten your back. With your left hand hold the back of an upright chair that is roughly at waist height. Extend your right foot forward about 60–90 cm (2–3 feet). Bend your right knee while dropping your left knee to the floor. Push back with your right knee and stabilize your position by holding the chair back throughout. Return to the start position. Finish your repetitions on this side, then switch over. Move the chair to your other side and repeat. Do not let your knee go over the front of your foot in the stress position.

Difficulty level – Programme 1

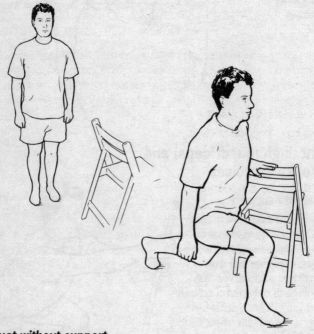

Squat without support

As for squat with support (see page 165), but start with hands by your side and raise them to the front when you squat for stability.

Difficulty level – Programme 2

Lunge without support

As for lunge with support (see above), but keep your hands by your side throughout.

Difficulty level – Programme 2

Buttocks and rear of thigh exercise

Lying back leg raise

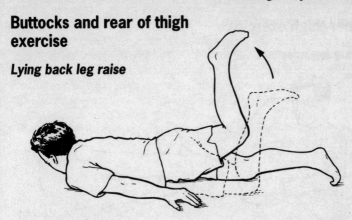

Lie face down on a mat with your palms down by your sides and your legs straight, 10 cm (4 inches) apart. Bend your left leg so the lower part points straight up. Now move your left knee 5–8 cm (2–3 inches) off the ground, hold for a brief moment then repeat. Once the repetitions are finished, change legs and repeat. Breathe in on the way up and out on the way down.

Difficulty level – Programmes 1 and 2

Hamstrings exercise

Back leg push

While kneeling on all fours on a mat, bring your left knee towards your left elbow, then fully extend the leg behind you. Hold briefly and repeat. Do not let the foot on the working leg touch the floor. Breathe in on the push up and out on the way down.

Difficulty level – Programmes 1 and 2

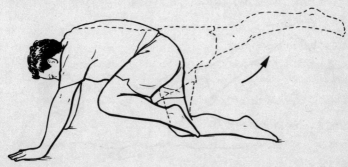

Inner thigh exercise

Lying leg raise

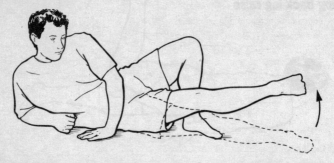

Lie on your side, with your top leg placed as shown and your foot flat on the floor. Raise your upper body on to your forearm, tighten your stomach, raise the straight leg and lower it under control. Repeat, then do the other side. Breathe in on the way up and out on the way down.

Difficulty level – Programmes 1 and 2

Outer thigh exercise

Side leg raise

Lie on your left side, with your right leg straight and your left leg bent. Point the toes of your right leg away from your body. Slowly lift your right leg up and then down. Do not let your pelvis move forward, but keep it in line with the rest of your body. Move your raised leg only to a height that can be controlled by your muscles. Do not swing the leg at any stage. Breathe in on the way up, out on the way down.

Difficulty level – Programmes 1 and 2

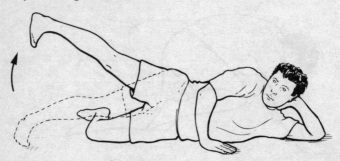

Calf exercises

Calf raise

Stand upright on the balls of your feet on a raised
platform no less than 7.5 cm (3 inches) high.
Lower your heels until you feel a good stretch, then
push up on your toes and raise your heels as high
as possible. Hold for a count of three, then repeat.
Breathe in on the way up, out on the way down.

Difficulty level – Programme 1

Single leg calf raise

Exactly the same exercise as the calf raise (above),
but use only one leg at a time. Tuck the foot of the
resting leg behind the ankle of the working one.

Difficulty level – Programme 2

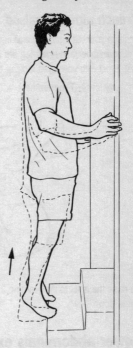

Upper abdominals exercises

Crunch

Lie on your back on a mat. Bend your knees and place your hands behind your head
with fingers intertwined. Pull in your stomach and flatten your lower back. Looking
straight up, press your head gently into the cup of your hands. Now lift, using your
upper abdominals to raise your shoulders from the ground. Maintain pressure with your
head in your hands and don't flick your elbows forward to gain momentum. Keep your
eyes on the ceiling. Once your shoulders are fully raised as far as they will naturally
go, slowly come back down. Breathe in on the way up and out on the way down.

Difficulty level – Programme 1

To raise the level to Programme 2, hold for one second at the top of the motion and
then come down slowly.

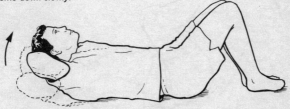

Crunch with legs raised

Position yourself against a wall in the position shown. Make sure your feet are crossed and your upper and lower leg are at 90 degrees to each other. Put your hands behind your head with your eyes looking at the ceiling. Repeat the motion as for the crunch.

Difficulty level – Programme 1

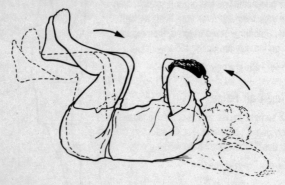

To raise the level to Programme 2, add a second at the top of the motion and then come down slowly.

Lower abdominals exercises

Reverse crunch

Lie face up on a mat with your hands resting on your lower abdominals. Pull your knees up to your chest, trying to lift your buttocks off the floor, and hold for a count of one. Return to the starting position. Do not arch your back at any stage of the exercise. Breathe in on the way up and out on the way down.

Difficulty level – Programmes 1 and 2

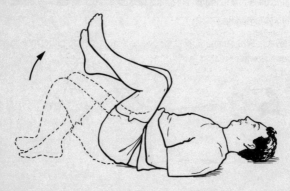

Alternate leg crunch

Lie on your back, with knees bent, feet flat on the floor and stomach pulled in. Place your hands, intertwined, behind your head and your elbows out at right angles from your body. Press your head gently into your hands and, using your abdominals, raise your shoulders off the ground. Keep your eyes on the ceiling. At the same time, lift your left leg off the ground and move your knee towards your forehead till it is approximately 15 cm (6 inches) away from it. Now slowly lower your leg and shoulders to the ground. Repeat the exercise using the other leg. Breathe in on the way up, out on the way down. Perform the exercise slowly.

Difficulty level – Programme 1

Raise it to Programme 2 by adding a second beat in the stress position.

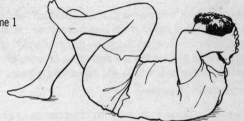

Oblique abdominals exercises

Side crunch

Lie face up on a mat with your legs bent and knees pointing to one side as shown in the picture. Ensure both shoulders are in contact with the ground. Place both hands, intertwined, behind your head. Gently push your head into your hands and look at the ceiling. Lift your shoulders from the ground as far as they naturally go and then lower yourself back to the first position under control. Repeat, then change sides. Breathe in on the way up, out on the down.

Difficulty level – Programme 1

It becomes Programme 2 if you add a second beat in the stress position.

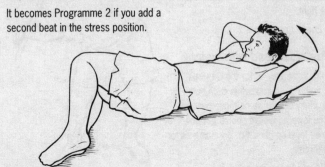

Crunch twist

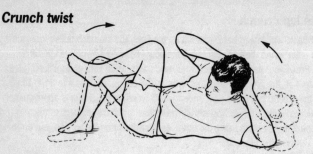

Lie on your back, with knees bent, feet flat, stomach pulled in and back flat. Place your hands behind your head with fingers intertwined. Pivoting on the left elbow (which stays on the floor) use your abdominals to raise your right elbow. At the same time, bring your left knee towards your right elbow. Once they touch over your stomach, hold briefly, then lower your leg and shoulder to the ground. Repeat, then swap sides.

Difficulty level – Programme 2

Make it more difficult by holding in the stress position for a second beat.

Outer obliques exercises

Standing side-bend with pole

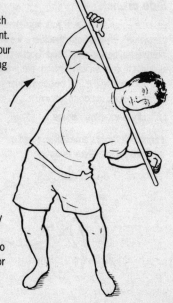

Stand with feet shoulders width apart, stomach pulled in, back flattened and knees slightly bent. Lay the pole across your shoulders and put your hands over it as shown in the diagram. Keeping your body in line, slowly bend over to the left and then to the right. Keep your knees bent and static. Breathe in whenever your body is rising and out every time it moves to the left or the right.

Difficulty level – Programme 1

Standing side-bend with weight

Stand in the same way as for the previous exercise. Holding a dumb-bell in each hand, by your side, carry out the same movement as before. The lowered weight should get down to around knee level on each dip. Breathing as for the last exercise.

Difficulty level – Programme 2

16
Further Training

When Richard trains actors for a specific film, his priority is to decide what the aim of the training actually is, what result is expected for the actor's body. Time tends to be limited, so the exercise programme is geared towards achieving the quickest, safest results, usually timed to coincide with the start of the film. He then tries to maintain the actor's fitness level throughout the duration of the film.

Maintenance is an important aspect of everyday training and overall health. People too often train, get a result and then fail to maintain it at a realistic level. They then have to repeat the whole initial training phase. For this reason, Richard generally encourages people to insert into their routine a circuit-training programme.

Circuit training

Circuit training combines the cardiovascular aspects of Zones 1 and 2 and the strength-training aspects of Programmes 1 and 2. It works the middle ground of fitness training. It doesn't burn as much fat as Zones 1 and 2 or build muscle as effectively as programmes 1 and 2, but it contains elements of both. This cuts down training time into one overall session and, because minimal equipment is required, it is ideal for training in a hotel room or at home.

How do I do circuit training?

For your circuit-training routine, we recommend that you do a series of strength-training exercises (like those in the strength-training menu in the previous chapter), interspersed with cardiovascular-type exercises such as jogging on the spot, skipping or stepping – anything that raises your heart rate to a level around 65 to 86 per cent of your Max HR. (A number of cardiovascular exercises are described at the end of the chapter.)

The strength-training exercises can also be organized to train the upper body first, then the lower body. For example, you can do one series of arm exercises, then switch to leg exercises. This will increase the demand on your heart to pump blood to the different areas being worked, because the muscles need extra fuel to function efficiently and carry away the waste material produced. This increased load on the heart is called peripheral heart action. It should be taken into account when you plan your overall body-training circuit programme.

Each set of circuit exercises of a strength-training or cardiovascular type should be carried out for between 20 and 60 seconds, with a 15-second rest between each set. If you are starting a training programme, the total circuit routine should last for 20 minutes. Increase the duration as your fitness level rises, up to a total of 60 minutes.

Strength-training exercises can be organized to give certain muscles a harder work-out than others. The slower-changing muscles in a problem area can be targeted in this way. You can even do a routine that consists entirely of exercises for lower-body muscle groups and really give that area an intense work-out. This should only be done when your strength and fitness levels can cope with that intensity of work, however. Similarly, you can load the exercises by doing more cardiovascular than strength exercises or vice versa to accent one part of your routine.

When should I do it?

Work circuit training into your routine once or twice a week to replace a full strength and cardiovascular routine. Duration, as we said before, depends on your fitness level, but start with a total of 20 minutes, with 20 seconds for each set. Increase both the duration and the weight or difficulty of the exercise as appropriate.

What equipment do I need?

A lot of the exercises we've suggested require no weights or special equipment. However, if you are away from home, maybe staying in a hotel without a gym, the following items could be of use:

- a skipping-rope
- an elastic resistance band to substitute for hand weights
- a short pole or chair for supported exercises

- a weight bench or low strong table
- a carpeted area or small mat
- a mirror to ensure correct form can be checked.

General circuit-training routine

The routine outlined in this section is designed to give equal emphasis to the strength-training and cardiovascular exercises.

- For the strength-training exercises, different muscle groups are identified (these are printed in *italics* in the list below). Choose an appropriate exercise for each group from the strength-training exercise menu in the previous chapter.

- The cardiovascular exercises (printed in plain type) can be found in the cardiovascular exercise menu on pages 176–177.

1. Star jumps
2. *Chest exercise*
3. Marching on the spot
4. *Front thigh and buttock exercise*
5. Skipping
6. *Shoulder exercise*
7. Shadow-boxing
8. *Triceps exercise*
9. Star jumps
10. *Hips exercise*
11. Marching on the spot
12. *Upper abdominals exercise*
13. Skipping
14. *Lower abdominals exercise*
15. Shadow-boxing
16. *Upper back exercise*
17. Star jumps
18. *Biceps exercise*
19. Marching on the spot
20. *Lower back exercise*
21. Skipping
22. *Buttocks and rear of thigh exercise*
23. Shadow-boxing
24. *Lower thigh exercise*

25. *Outer thigh exercise*
26. *Calves exercise*
27. Star jumps
28. Star jumps
29. *Oblique abdominal exercise*
30. *Outer oblique exercise*

Duration

If you spend 20 seconds on each exercise with 15 seconds' rest in between each set, the circuit will take about 17 minutes. If you spend 60 seconds on each exercise, again with 15 seconds' rest in between, the circuit will take about 37 minutes. Add 15 minutes for warming up and cooling down and stretching.

Cardiovascular exercise menu

- star jumps
- marching on the spot
- skipping (or simulated skipping)
- shadow-boxing (pretend to box, or get a punch bag).

Star jumps

Stand upright, feet together and hands by your side. Jump your legs outwards so they are about twice shoulder width apart. At the same time, bring your hands up in an arching motion to meet above your head. Reverse the motion back to the standing position. Bend your knees every time your feet land to cushion the impact. Repeat rhythmically over the period of exercise.

Marching on the spot

March, but in an exaggerated manner. Pump your arms and lift your knees so that the tops of your thighs brush your abdomen. Keep your head up, looking straight ahead at all times. (You might feel a bit of an idiot!)

Skipping

Skipping takes many forms and is a skill that needs to be practised. Buy a rope and work your way into it slowly. If you find it doesn't get better, forget the rope and perform a running motion instead, making skipping motions with your hands and lower arms. If you feel silly remember that boxers do it all the time and it's good exercise.

Shadow-boxing

Get in front of a mirror and pretend your reflection is your opponent. Flick punches on to their chin and other target areas. Remember to move your feet around as well. You should be doing this quite fast, so that your heart rate is elevated. Experiment with different punches. If you find this difficult, buy a boxing video and study it or go to a local boxercise class to learn the different punch combinations.

17
We Go Playing

When I started this course I was probably more unfit than most of the people who will read this book. And now I am fit. The next chapter deals with some of the extreme things that I did on the way to getting to where I am now. But let's make this clear: we don't expect you to do any of them. I did them because I wanted to and sometimes just because I could. I have gone further down the line than I expect you to because I wanted to see just how fit I could get.

We set several goals on the path to finishing at my ideal weight. First I had to ride a bicycle to Brighton, swim 2400 metres (1¹/₂ miles) in the cold November sea, and then ride back to London the next day. Then I had to do a free-fall parachute jump. Finally, we walked up Pen-y-fan mountain in Wales. (This mountain is used for training the English Special Forces and it's tough on walkers.)

The distance between London and Brighton is approximately 88.5 kilometres (55 miles), and the route is hilly to say the least. It is the venue for an annual cycle race where the winners complete the distance in something like two and a half hours. But they do it on road bikes, all the traffic is stopped for them and they are extremely fit. We decided to do it a more leisurely pace.

We started at ten o'clock one Friday morning from Streatham. I had packed a back-pack with my toothbrush, camera, swimming costume, wallet and a bottle of aftershave. (Why the aftershave I have no idea.) The first few kilometres were fine and slipped by quickly.

One last piece of advice: buy or borrow some sort of personal stereo, because it makes the time go more quickly. One of the truths that fit people hide from you is that exercise is very boring indeed. But if you have a radio or a Walkman it helps to speed up the time. This is especially true on a running machine.

Richard decided to stop every hour and, to my great delight, on the first stop we bought some energy bars. When you are going to do hard exercise over a couple of hours you need to replace stored energy calories, otherwise you come to a grinding halt. I felt a childish delight in stuffing these calories into my body. The third hour was much harder and my back began to ache from the shoulder-straps of my pack.

By now I was feeling really tired. During the course of my training I had been surreptitiously measuring my fitness against Richard's. On this exercise it became apparent that Richard was about 700 times fitter than I was, even in my improved state.

Then it happened: I got a flat tyre. Richard had told me to be sure to get a spare inner tube in case we had a flat tyre, and in fact I had been forced to abandon a previous solo attempt due to a flat tyre, so I should have remembered to include this vital piece of equipment. But I forgot it all the same. This meant that I had to use Richard's spare inner tube.

The third hour passed in a kind of dream. My body had given up on any kind of feeling and just continued to work without any thought. The fourth hour was better because the end of the journey was in sight. Then we finished the sweets and the last hour was hell.

We arrived in Brighton feeling very pleased with ourselves and went down to the sea for the second half of the exercise: the swim. I had decided that I was too bloody tired to do it, but Richard was being all Special Forces about it. I wandered down to the edge of the shore hoping that he would get struck by lightning or get a heart attack or something. As it happened, I nearly got my wish.

That sea was the coldest water I've ever been in and we had to start swimming fairly vigorously just to keep warm. For the first half we were swimming with the tide and everything was fine. But as we turned round to come back, Richard got cramp really badly. We were now swimming against a fast-flowing tide about 800 metres (half a mile) out from the shore. Richard was getting worse. His legs had stopped working properly, so he swam for safety as best he could. I decided to carry on, because I was determined to finish the course. In the end, the tide just got too strong for me to continue, but I managed to swim very nearly back to where we had started, thus securing a moral victory.

Our journey back was a rerun of the journey down, except that about 11 km (7 miles) out of Horsham it was Richard's turn to get a flat and, because I had used his spare the day before, we couldn't change it. Without saying a word Richard picked up his bike and ran all the way to Horsham, albeit rather tight-lipped. This highlights an important lesson, which is that if you're embarking on an adventure where you're relying on your equipment, check it prior to starting and keep checking it throughout.

Free-fall parachuting

Richard had also planned for us both to do a free-fall parachute jump with the help of his mates in the Red Devils Parachute team. But when the time came, he had to go to Russia to train Julia Ormond and so I went on my own.

The Joint Services Parachute centre is in Netheravon, Salisbury. The idea – as discussed in the pub – was that I would do a 3800-metre (12,500-foot) free-fall parachute jump and at the same time get my picture taken for *GQ* magazine, for whom we were writing an article.

Army camps all over the world have a certain bleakness about them. A depressed-looking guard examines your pass and eventually lifts the barrier to let you into the camp, after giving you directions and warning you not to get lost. You then get lost, because his directions would confuse a homing pigeon, and all the buildings look exactly the same. When I finally found the canteen, I was greeted by the sight of a bunch of twenty-year-old, incredibly fit-looking paratroopers consuming roughly 8 million calories of breakfast each (the bastards).

A year before this I had enquired about the chance of doing a parachute jump at a civilian club. I was told that I was too fat and too old. If you are over 40, you need a doctor's certificate to say that you are fit enough to hurl yourself out of an aeroplane, and you should really weigh under 100 kilos (16 stone) for normal jumping.

My instructor was called Jason Grimes and he was the survivor of over 3000 jumps. He was going to teach me on a one-to-one basis and at the end of the day I would jump out of a plane with a paratrooper holding on to each leg. Then I would free-fall to 1500 metres (5000 feet), pull my rip-cord and glide gracefully to the landing point. At this stage I wasn't at all nervous and felt that I would be a natural.

We started the lecture. 'I will give you knowledge, because knowledge dispels fear,' Jason stated. We watched a video showing all of the things that could go wrong with a jump. I suspect that this is the first weeding-out process. If you can watch all those tangled parachutes plummeting to earth and still fail to make the connection with what you're doing, you may just be stupid enough actually to do the jump.

I was worried that you had to be fantastically fit to do this, but it's more a question of nerve than fitness. During the morning we listened to various lectures and we learnt the parts of the parachute. This was a bit unnerving, because there are a fair few of them and they sort of interact to let the parachute go.

At lunch I had two white cheese rolls with no butter. This is what we mean by minimizing the damage. In a place where nobody needs to lose weight and everything is picked for its positive calorific content, you are pushed to find anything that could be regarded as low calorie. So you just lose whatever calories you can. Drink Diet Coke instead of the full version. Drop butter from the roll. It's small stuff but it all helps.

After lunch we went to the gym to learn about how we should behave diving towards the earth. When you fall through the sky, you have to push your pelvis forward and your arms and your legs backwards. This is quite hard to do and the position is one that requires a certain amount of suppleness. Certainly you have to be reasonably fit to do it.

The actual jumping part first seemed real when we walked out to the aeroplane that was to be our launching platform. As we sat on the edge of the door through which we would later jump, I had a sudden premonition of what the jump would be like and I wasn't too comfortable with the idea. I half considered not doing it although I knew that, come hell or high water, I would go through with it.

'Does anyone ever refuse to jump?' I asked Jason. He gave me the most evil grin I have ever seen one human being give another. 'Not once we've got them in the plane, no sir,' he said.

We went over to the briefing room to get a flight time and discovered that there was a low cloud base, which meant that there would be no jumping that day. I wasn't sure whether to feel elated or disappointed. On the whole I would rather have got it out of the way quickly. This way I had to go through the process of getting brave all over again.

Several days later the same gloomy guard looked at my pass and waved me into the camp. The same café was playing host to a different set of young paratroopers eating for England.

Because it was some days since my original training, I had to retrain. At this point the weather was again a bit uncertain, with a low cloud base, so there was still some doubt about whether we would go. In the gym we went back through the complicated procedures that I would follow once I left the plane. 'But,' said Jason, 'the most important thing to remember is always to obey the jump master. That's me.'

Here is the theory of how free-fall parachuting works. You have two people who jump with you and they hold on to the leg of your jumpsuit. (There are two of them in case one of the instructors blacks out, in which case the other will get you down safely.) As you fall, you have to scan the horizon to make sure you are more or less the right way up and check your height using your wrist altimeter. You then relay the information to both instructors, one at a time. At this point you practise locating the rip-cord that releases your parachute. You do this three times. Then you do another scan and again inform your instructors of your height. By this time you have fallen to around 1800 metres (6000 feet). At 1670 metres (5500 feet) you put your thumb and forefinger together to indicate that you are in 'the circle of awareness'. You flash your fingers twice to inform both instructors that you are at 1500 metres (5000 feet) and then you reach back and pull your rip-cord. All this takes about 40 seconds, so you have to be fast.

At two o'clock that afternoon it was decided that we would be going jumping. We clambered into the plane, some, it must be said, more willingly than others. My instructors and I sat at the front of the plane, because we were to be the last out. It took 25 minutes for the plane to climb to the required height for our free fall and there was so much noise that you couldn't talk. But you could think.

At 900 metres (3000 feet) several of the other people in the plane left to do a line jump. This involves simply getting out of the plane and waiting for the parachute to open automatically. How I envied them their relatively easy task.

At last we reached a height of 3600 metres (12,000 feet). I couldn't see the ground, because it was covered in a thick blanket of cloud, but I assumed it was there. I moved to the edge of the plane and crouched ready to do the check-out manoeuvre that precedes the jump. It is difficult to explain my feelings at that moment. There was terror, but there was also a grim acceptance of the inevitability of the situation. The men jumping with me were Red Devils and it would have been unthinkable to bottle out of the jump. My worst nightmare was that the whole camp would know within minutes that I had failed; nothing moves faster in a services environment than gossip about failure.

Finally, crouched in the howling of the wind on the edge of that aeroplane over 3 kilometres (2 miles) above Salisbury Plain, the moment had arrived for me to launch myself out into – nothing. I did the checks and threw myself out too quickly so as not to allow myself to fail.

The sensation of leaving that plane was amazing. The whole world exploded into a blaze of white and the noise was phenomenal. My face started flapping and felt as if it were being pushed backwards. It took me valuable seconds to realign myself and to remember that the world was coming up to meet me at over 190 kph (120 mph). I started going through the drills, but because of the time I had spent being overawed, I couldn't complete all of them.

There was a sudden jerk, I had a feeling of complete disorientation and I realized that Jason had pulled my rip-cord and I was floating under my canopy. The sudden shock of stopping had, however, caused my goggles to fill with water. The male reproductive organs were not designed to decelerate from over 160 kph (100 mph) to slightly less than 30 kph (20 mph) in less than 100 metres. I had to take my hands off of the steering lines and empty my goggles to avoid drowning at 1500 metres (5000 feet).

There was a sudden splendid moment when I realized that I had made the jump, my parachute had opened and that I had a story that I could use in the pub for ever. But there was still the small matter of the remaining 1200 metres (4000 feet) to the ground. I moved left and right as I had been instructed to do. The thing about parachuting is that they tell you what it's going to be like, but after that it's very much up to you. You are on your own journey of discovery.

I flared out a bit too late and landed in a slightly undignified heap on the ground. But I was down, and with all the limbs I had started the day with. And the most amazing feeling of achievement. Every sensation was magnified, each sense working slower so that I could savour everything to the full. That moment made all the exercise, all the work and all the struggles to avoid fatty foods worthwhile.

Mountaineering in Wales

We had to do one more exercise to satisfy Richard's blood lust. Courtesy of one of his old sergeants, we were to climb Pen-y-fan in Wales under strict supervision. Brian Bosley now runs an outdoor adventure training company known as Outer Limits. After 17 years of teaching paratroopers physical fitness, his love of the mountains was so ingrained that he could not leave them. So he decided to rent out his considerable expertise to civilians.

We arrived in Wales feeling pretty ropy after enduring traffic jams all the way down the M4. The plan was that we would climb to the top of the mountain, wait for sunrise and then come back down. We had a third member of the party, James, who is the holder of five different black belts and one of the fittest people I had ever met.

I was frightened about this exercise for three reasons: one, it was snowing and the side of the mountain was around a metre (3 feet) deep in snow; two, these were very serious men indeed and I was scared of letting myself down, and, three, I didn't want to put the other members of the party at risk.

It worked out fine, however, because Richard had prepared me better than I thought. We had to climb solidly for two and a half hours through the deep snow, but it was rewarding to be part of a team working together to achieve something. We made the top around half an hour before sunrise. The most nerve-racking part was a pass that we had to cross with a 1800-metre (2800-foot) drop to our left.

When we got to the top we made a cup of tea and climbed into our sleeping-bags to watch the sun come up. It was truly one of the most magnificent sights I have ever seen. A perfect day was developing, with stunning visibility.

All of a sudden our guide, Gled Gledhill, jumped up and said, 'Right, I want everybody moving right now.' I thought he was joking, as we has been taking the mickey out of each other all morning. But the serious expression on Richard's face made me instinctively jump up and follow the others as they broke into a run. By the time we reached the dangerous pass about 20 minutes later, you couldn't see your hand in front of your face, the temperature had dropped alarmingly and the mountain seemed like a very dangerous place.

We made it safely down, but later we heard that someone had died on the same part of the mountain that day.

As a finale to the weekend, I was to try abseiling. I didn't want to, because I was tired and I was scared. I had also unaccountably developed vertigo for the first time in my life. I climbed very unwillingly to the top of the 36-metre (120-foot) cliff from which I would launch myself into thin air on a piece of rope thinner than my finger. I did it, but it was terrifying because there are basically two bits of ground that can hurt you: the one in front of you and the one below. I'm not quite sure how I got to the bottom, but somehow I did.

Richard came up and asked what I thought. 'I bloody hate it,' I said. 'Right, up again,' he said and to my intense surprise I found myself climbing up again wondering how he had managed to make me do it.

The second time it was more controlled but I still felt it was not for me. 'How was it?' Richard asked. 'No better,' I replied, truthfully if stupidly. 'Right, up again,' he said.

By this time I had worked out the least painful way up the hill and the run down was also easier. 'Better?' asked Richard. I braved it out. 'No, Richard, I really bloody hate abseiling.' 'Yes,' he said, 'so do I.'

Arctic exercise

I also gave my heart a severe testing without meaning to, as you will see from the following, an article I wrote for *GQ* magazine:

Nothing works properly in the Arctic Circle. Batteries discharge in seconds rather than hours, clothes become solid in minutes if not worn. Warmer is worse than cold because the snow becomes unstable and very dangerous. But the climate, the harshest known to man, is considered to be very good for Royal Marines.

A thousand miles north of Oslo a long-haired Norwegian conscript raises a lethargic wave as we drive through the gates into the Asegarden army barracks. The camp has been taken over by the cold-weather training arm of the Royal Marines. Treacherous-looking paths are carved through snow which is higher than head height. The first night we are not allowed to leave the hut in case we die before we have had the mandatory cold-weather survival lecture. The lecture is delivered in Geordie monotone by one of the mountain specialists. It contains advice such as, 'If you get caught in an avalanche, dribble. Note which way the spit moves so you can work out which way up you are.' Then we sit through slides warning of the perils of frostbite. A hint here: if you get infected bits don't rush to the nearest fire because, and this is important, you have to raise the core body temperature.

And on the subject of the inner man, these Marines eat an amazing amount. Most of us eat around 2000 calories a day. Someone involved in heavy physical exercise uses about 3500. A normal Army ration for this environment contains 8000 calories a day. Canteen chips and creamy cakes are the norm. Survival is a hard business this far north and the body needs as many calories as it can get to fuel the monotonous but essential fight against the incredibly pervasive cold. The Royal Marines don't stop operating in the field until the temperature drops to minus 30 centigrade. To put that into perspective, the average temperature in a domestic freezer is minus 20 centigrade.

You are repeatedly told not to touch anything metal with your bare skin. An odd but frequent injury is that people lick the end of their ski poles, which have tiny metal screws in. They get lectures telling them not to, they get specifically warned about this and yet they still do it because they can't believe it's really dangerous. But it is and it hurts when you have to rip off the flesh in your tongue to release yourself, apparently.

One of the main reasons that I have come here is to do an ice jump. This gives the soldiers an experience of what happens when you are crossing frozen lakes and are unlucky enough to fall in. This makes them very careful when crossing frozen lakes in the future.

We gather to start the exercise. Twenty-seven of us are all dressed identically in T-shirts, tracksuit bottoms and a very thin white polythene suit called Cam Whites. There is a faintly kamikaze air about the whole proceedings. We huddle in the shelter of the BV 206 snow vehicles to listen to a lecture from Bob Colville, the Royal Marines' most senior and respected mountain leader. Everyone is joking rather nervously. 'Now I want to explain the procedures that we use to get you a thousand miles to hospital in Oslo if you fuck this up,' he says laconically. There is immediately the deepest and most respectful silence that I have ever heard.

We walk to the lake to watch the demonstration. There is a hole about 20 feet by 12 cut into the ice. The wind howls across miles of desolate whiteness, it's bitterly cold and relentlessly noisy. The Royal Marine Sergeant demonstrating puts on his skis, picks up a back pack and falls agonizingly slowly into the icy water. He's got a horrible hangover, he was the jolliest of us all in the bar last night. He has to get the pack, containing 5 gallons of water in a jerrycan, out before he can get out. He has several goes and is struggling. He makes it out of the water and rolls in the snow to get warm before being whisked away to get changed in the vehicle.

I am the only civilian doing this, I am the only person over thirty and I'm terrified of making a complete arse of myself in a situation where the blokes have little else to talk about. It comes to my turn. I pick up the pack and loop it over one shoulder. This is the way that mountaineers carry packs in dangerous conditions so that they can throw them away and save themselves. I hit the water after being pushed hard from behind. As my head goes underwater I can just hear the tail end of the question 'Are you ready?' obviously uttered just after I'd been pushed. There are about twenty words in the English language to describe variants of cold. But none of them describe this sensation. It is mind-blowingly, heart-stoppingly cold.

I manage to find the pack, swim to the edge of the ice and on my fifth go I get it over and on to the edge. Make no mistake here, the pack comes out or you don't. And it's not light, the jerrycan is filled with 5 gallons of water, remember. Then I find the ski poles and use them as daggers to pull myself out. I have been in the water only 18 seconds. As I run back to the snow tractor, I begin to slow down. I can feel the energy draining out of my body and I have an almost comic sense of watching myself from outside. If that had happened in the water it would have been dangerous, to say the least.

In the armed services you are excused this exercise over the age of forty on the grounds that it is dangerous for your heart.

As I said at the beginning of this chapter, to undertake all the things that I did during the period after I got fit is not a course of action that we are recommending to you, nor is it in any way mandatory. For me, as a 43-year-old bloke, to be able to achieve these goals was an amazing sensation. But you reach a point where you are reasonably fit and as healthy as you are going to get and there is no longer any correlation between the two. For example, Linford Christie is a lot fitter than I am, but he may not be a lot healthier. Sometimes the pressures under which athletes put their bodies are detrimental to them. The most important thing is that you use your new fitness for your pleasure. You may find that you like running or cycling; I did to my surprise. It's about fun and about feeling better in yourself. It's for your benefit.

Index